Eddie Brocklesby is the oldest British woman to have completed an Ironman triathlon, at the age of seventy-four. She has spent the last twenty years taking part in marathons, triathlons and Ironman races across the globe, has represented Great Britain in many European and World triathlon and duathlon championships, and cycled in a relay of over three thousand miles across America.

Eddie is passionate about the fitness of our ageing population, and founded the charity Silverfit in 2013 to organise fitness classes for older people. The charity and Eddie's sporting achievements have garnered much national attention in the media.

IRONGRAN

How keeping fit taught me
that growing older needn't
mean slowing down

EDWINA
BROCKLESBY

sphere

SPHERE

First published in Great Britain in 2018 by Sphere

1 3 5 7 9 10 8 6 4 2

A CIP catalogue record for this book
is available from the British Library.

ISBN 978-0-7515-7111-0

Typeset in Bembo by M Rules
Printed and bound in Great Britain by
Clays Ltd, St Ives plc

Papers used by Sphere are from well-managed forests
and other responsible sources.

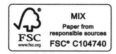

Sphere
An imprint of
Little, Brown Book Group
Carmelite House
50 Victoria Embankment
London EC4Y 0DZ

An Hachette UK Company
www.hachette.co.uk

www.littlebrown.co.uk

I dedicate this book to the ultimate relay:
To my beloved late husband for our shared times
together and for continuing to inspire me today, and to
my children for enthusiastically accepting the baton in
encouraging me to live life to the full.

CONTENTS

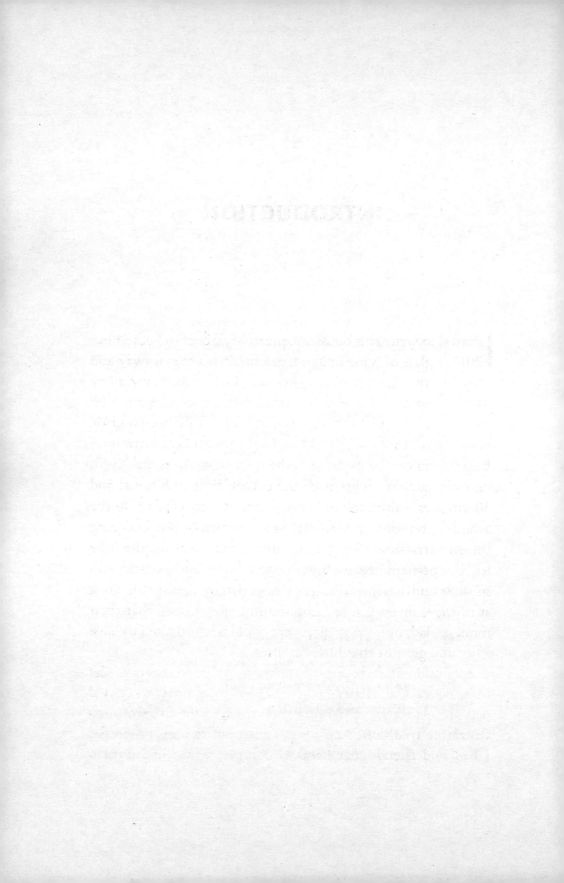

INTRODUCTION

I started to write this book in Lanzarote airport in September 2014, a glass of wine in hand, gazing across the runway and planes to the Atlantic Ocean beyond. I had come over a few days earlier to do a Half Ironman, which involved a 1.9k swim in a beautiful salty lagoon, 90k of a hilly but fantastic bike ride and a painfully hot and very tough half marathon. I had stood on the podium as the only woman in the 70–74 year old category who made the cut-off time of 8 hours and 30 minutes – although only just. They had cheered me at the awards ceremony in Club La Santa, probably not knowing the embarrassingly long, long time I had spent on the bike leg, but perhaps because I was seventy-one, enthusiastic, still smiling and having fun. They hoped they could still do it at my age, or even more importantly, they hoped that their mum or dad, or even grandparent could be motivated to have a go, and get just that little bit fitter.

Alongside that happy memory, as I gazed beyond the runway, was fear. Between the sea and me was a narrow coastal path. It forms part of the marathon route of the full Ironman Lanzarote triathlon. And I was signed up. In a rash moment I had told friends that I would compete again in Ironman

Lanzarote. I had done the race three times before but then I had been in my sixties. Now I was over seventy, it was different. I watched from the window as my red bike box was towed to the plane. What on earth motivates me, at my advancing age – and with two problematic knees – to aim to do another Ironman? I knew I faced fifteen to twenty hours of training every week for a year, much of it alone, most of it in the slow lane of the swimming pool, or long solo bike rides in the Surrey Hills, and limited running to minimise the stress on my knees. Yet I reflected that if my story could make a difference to just a few people, inspire them to be more active and reduce the cost to the NHS and social care, and help build a happier, healthier ageing population, then it would be worth it.

I often hear that I am inspirational. I'm told 'You don't look or act seventy-five', 'I hope I can do it when I am your age', and the heartbreaking 'I wish *my* mum . . .' It's lovely and flattering to be told that you are inspirational, but does anyone believe they really are?

So here follows a reflection on my life. It has been fascinating to look back. What struck me was that in my fifty years of social work, I have never deviated far from the belief that life is 80:20 nurture versus nature. Genetics plays a role, but those crucial nine months *in utero* and then after birth – the love, care and support of those around you – give you your true start in life. Understanding that can help us support the next generation better.

I only started running at the age of fifty. I came to love group runs, and the peace, fresh air and joy of those long, long runs on my own. Running helped me through the crisis points in my own life. When my husband of thirty years died, I knew I was the lucky one as we had just enough time to share our feelings, and he was able, without anger, to give me permission to go on to enjoy life.

Physical activities such as running, walking, biking and even swimming have given me incredible social outlets and opportunities to give something back. There is so much emphasis these days on our ageing population, whose increasingly complex needs are a burden on the NHS.

So this is an opportune moment to reflect on my life, my hopes and how I can use my allegedly inspirational, legendary and probably crazy status of being an Irongran to make a difference to our ageing, sedentary population. Having helped to set up the Silverfit charity, with an aim to promote physical activity and socialising for older people, can I somehow add to, or increase, the public awareness of the massive weight of evidence that physical activity is not only good for you, it is vital for our economy, NHS and social-care system. And our survival as happy, healthy oldies means we are able to continue to contribute to society rather than cost a fortune in social care. Physical inactivity is the greatest killer, and precursor of illness, dependency and unhealthy ageing.

If I can move, despite my osteoarthritic knees, from starting to run at fifty to my first small triathlon in my sixties to being, at seventy-four, the oldest British woman to complete an Ironman, having so much fun en route, I hope you will realise that it is never too late to start exercising, having fun and being SILVERFIT!

1

Staying healthy isn't rocket science

One of my favourite and best rules that I have come to live by is *Don't eat anything your grandmother wouldn't recognise,* although I'm not sure this rule applies directly to me as my grandmother was a bit different. Georgina Landemare – Nan to me – was Winston and Clementine Churchill's personal cook for fifteen years, throughout and after the war. She had a powerful influence on me, with her positive attitude towards life, her enthusiasm, compassion, energy and constant sense of fun. Only as I helped the Imperial War Museum to publish *Churchill's Cookbook,* a reissue of *Recipes from No. 10,* the Anglo-French cookery book she had written in 1958, to excellent newspaper reviews, did I have the chance to explore her history and reflect on her impact on my mother, as her only child, and indeed myself.

Painstakingly, by hand, Nan started to write her auto-biography at the age of ninety-five. It started with 'To my son-in-law, who always talks about the bad old days'. She then recounted her happy experiences as the oldest child of a coachman and his wife, who often had to take responsibility for her younger siblings. She recalled the relative poverty in which they lived but the richness of family life growing up in rural Buckinghamshire, living on plain basic food that was always fresh and locally produced. She used to go and stay with her aunt who she described as interested in cooking, with a healthy stock-pot always on the go.

Aged fourteen, Nan started to work as a scullery maid in a family home, with the responsibility for cleaning coppers. Later in her life she gave her copper saucepans to me, insisting that I must regularly get them re-tinned as the copper was poisonous.

It was while working as a scullery maid at the Ritz that Nan met Paul Landemare, the French head chef at the hotel. He had come from a family home in Paris, and his own father was a patissier. Nan used to insist that my grandfather had invented the macaron, but the internet suggests they originated with Italian nuns. Paul was married to Annette, and they had five children. Family mythology reports a fight with knives in the kitchens between Paul and Annette. In 1909, at the age of fifty-seven, Annette died of cancer and barely two months later Paul married Georgina, twenty-three years his junior.

One day, towards the end of her life, I went into Nan's room, and found her tearing up a sheaf of handwritten notes and putting the shreds down the plughole of her small corner sink. She told me it was her autobiography, a book my mother had said no one would be interested in it. I grabbed it from her and saved nineteen pages detailing her early childhood. What history was lost down that plughole?

I remain unclear about the years from 1932 to 1939, but Nan rose from being a scullery maid to become an amazingly successful woman in the male-dominated world of chefs. According to Clementine Churchill's diary, Nan cooked for Winston and Clementine Churchill at Newmarket races,

Cowes, debutante balls and more: Nan always said she had cooked for sixteen kings, although no one has been able to name them for me. Hopefully Annie Gray, who is writing a biography of Nan, will be able to fill in some of those gaps. She organised huge dinners and banquets, and made many close friends, including Sir Ian Hamilton, Churchill's close companion in the 18890s North West Frontier war. (She wrote to me once: 'General Sir Ian Hamilton always asked to see me whenever he came to No 10, and he left me the sunray clock in his will.') When I met Lady Soames, Winston and Clementine's youngest daughter Mary, she told me that her parents could only occasionally afford to have Nan cook for them at Chartwell over a weekend.

Nan was fifty-eight years old when war broke out in 1939. Clementine Churchill's diary records a visit from Nan on 5 January 1940 to offer her full-time services to the Churchill family, as her war effort. It was an offer that was gratefully accepted. She remained with them for fifteen years, in and out of No 10 Downing Street, and finally at their home in Hyde Park Gate. Visiting her there as a child, I remember so clearly walking with her to see the nearby Peter Pan statue that J. M. Barrie had commissioned in Kensington Gardens.

On 14 October 1940, during an air raid, Churchill had instructed the staff at No 10 to go down to the basement for shelter. Nan had delayed her departure, apparently too immersed in the crucial task of cooking the mousseline pudding. Fortunately, Winston Churchill came into the kitchen and insisted she went down to the shelter with him. He rescued her just in time: three minutes later the very spot where they had both been standing became a scene of complete devastation. I nearly lost my grandmother and the country their prime minister.

*

My mother Yvonne was born and christened in Pimlico in 1915, and although the family home remained there she recalled a childhood of moving from one house to another with her parents' work. It is only with hindsight that I realise how little I know about Mum's past, or her depression, which I know surfaced from time to time.

Mum met my father, seven years her senior, when they were both students at Morley College, in Lambeth, in the thirties. Dad, a writer and cricketer with far-left views, was far from seeing eye to eye with any of Nan's aristocratic and conservative friends. He had been editor of the college's magazine for three years when, in 1939, he was awarded an English Speaking Union Scholarship to the United States. He returned to Morley College with material for their magazine, and opposed to the war. Of that time, he later wrote:

'I think we saw Morley appropriately as a college for working men and women and we wrote and spoke and acted accordingly. There was trouble at the time of Munich; that editorial had stung a person in very high places indeed' – and from then Dad wrote that 'the editor said his political pieces under a by line. He was very nearly right about Munich! All this was in the days when opinion stood for something more than a digit in a Gallup Poll.'

Dad's own editorship 'ended abruptly – the issue was all but ready for Sept 1939. There was a faint air of martyrdom about it but the writers were eventually excused the firing line. Instead as the days were counted down to September 3rd we filled sandbags and stacked them around the gymnasium windows, and on the day we joined George Cottrell in charge of about fifteen hundred indignant mothers, expectant mothers and children who were being evacuated from Bermondsey.'

Dad was employed within the National Association of Boys' Clubs in 1940 and remained there till his retirement.

He wrote many plays for the BBC, and several novels and pamphlets. An intelligent, charismatic, optimistic, thoughtful and highly creative and articulate person, with a great sense of fun, Dad had a profound influence on me.

My parents married in the Catholic church at Chiswick in 1939 and they moved to Nottingham where, as a key worker, Dad avoided being called up. A few years later they moved to Bristol, where I was born in 1943. I still have a card on No 10 embossed headed card, addressed to my grandmother: 'For your little granddaughter with good wishes for her future, Clementine Churchill.' And on the back is a reference to a matinee jacket she had sent to me.

I grew up in Bristol. From time to time, my father and I would go down to Temple Meads to meet Nan off the London train. She was a warm, plump and cuddly figure, delighted and excited to come to stay with us. Despite it being an era of stringent rationing, she always carried interesting parcels. Butter, Italian Amaretto biscuits and fresh produce from the Chartwell farm arrived, and unusual presents like the delightful money box the carpenter at No 10 had made for me from one of Churchill's cigar boxes.

The contrast for Nan must have been huge. She would leave the glitz of the celebrity lifestyle – the heroes, the royalty and the Chiefs of Staff for whom she was cooking – to come down to Bristol to be 'just a nan'.

Nan was profoundly shocked when Churchill lost the July 1945 election and the family moved out of No 10. In 1973, she was tearful when she described to Joan Bakewell, on BBC Television's *Times Remembered: Below Stairs*, Labour's landslide victory as 'the wish of the soldiers'. When Churchill returned to Downing Street after six years out of office, Nan described the warmth of the welcome she received from all the staff at No 10, and even the police guarding Downing

Street. Now, I watch Nan in that memorable BBC interview on her ninety-first birthday, surrounded by telegrams
including Lady Churchill's, and recall her anger when Lord
Moran published his book revealing Churchill's history of
ill health. Nan knew, from her own experiences, and those
of the many close friends still working with the family, how
unwell Churchill had been for many years before his death,
and how this information had been concealed from the
public. She went to see Churchill lying in state and attended
his funeral at St Paul's Cathedral in 1965. I still have the card
that shows her seat – South Aisle, Row C. Years later, I took
her up to Bladon, near Blenheim, to visit his simple grave. It
was a very moving experience.

I remember journeying up to see Nan in London several
times a year. We would stop in the car on the perimeter road
of the airport, so close to the runway, to watch the planes at
the tiny Heathrow aerodrome before visiting her either at 10
Downing Street or at 28 Hyde Park Gate. I remember sitting
in Churchill's chair in the Cabinet Room of No 10 in 1952,
when I was nine.

Nan's pride and the closeness and deep affection towards
Mrs Churchill stand out most vividly in my memory. Nan
was undoubtedly her close friend and confidante. Most
mornings, they had long get-togethers where guests were
discussed, menus were decided and preparations were made
for last-minute guests. Nothing fazed my grandmother, and
although Mrs Churchill was much feted for organising dinners for large numbers at very short notice, she relied heavily
on Nan to fulfil the promises and prepare the elaborate dinners for such historic meetings.

Nan was always full of energy and needed little sleep – one
of those genetic factors I seem to have inherited. She told me

she never went to bed until after Mr Churchill's last whisky, and she was up and ready to cook his breakfast at half-past eight every morning. And she didn't have the benefit of his famous after-lunch snooze. Churchill's personal secretary Elizabeth Nel told me how he had insisted on taking Nan out onto the balcony to see the crowds in Whitehall on VE Day. He thanked her, saying that without her efforts in looking after him, he could not have achieved this.

Nan must have been an incredibly organised and method-ical professional. When I met her in 2013, Lady Soames described to me her own deep fondness for Nan. She told me that even when she was responsible for huge banquets, Nan would be so organised that she would be sitting down doing a crossword or studying the horse-racing odds by the time the meal was ready to serve. Neither nature nor nurture has equipped me thus.

Mrs Churchill used to send me a book every Christmas but I never viewed it as anything other than just another book. I remember taking a copy of *Black Beauty* into school – 'To Edwina from Clementine Churchill', it said on a front page. At ten years old, I was rather surprised by the responses of the teachers – up until that time the Churchills were just Nan's employers and I hadn't really appreciated their significance. Interestingly, meeting with my school friends recently, they remembered more readily that Joan and Jackie Collins were my step-cousins – my father's stepmother was their pater-nal aunt.

In 1954 Nan finally retired, aged seventy-two. By then, she was seriously overweight, which she put down to tasting all those creamy soups. She was on a range of medication for heart troubles but after a diagnosis of diverticulitis she was taken off all medication and put on a high-fibre diet. She lost all the excess weight, and as proof that it is never too late to change your lifestyle, she lived for a further fifteen healthy years.

She led a remarkably independent life – cooking for herself, receiving loads of visitors, writing hundreds of letters and long, long lists of Christmas cards sent and received. She was a devoted grandmother and wonderful great-grandmother, with an endless supply of brittle-nut toffee and welcome silver coins whenever we visited.

Lady Churchill had inspired and encouraged Nan to write *Recipes from No 10*. My mother laboriously typed them all out from handwritten notes, and I well remember my mother's difficulties in persuading Nan to translate some of her directions, such as for 'handfuls of flour', into pounds and ounces. It was a long, arduous task, and after one review by the publisher the typewritten notes were passed to Lady Churchill, who wrote the foreword. Lady Churchill then went through the publisher's proof, putting in the French accents and adding the necessary plurals. Fascinatingly, in her initial foreword, Lady Churchill referred to 'housewives', but the publisher changed this to 'her readers': 'Mrs Landemare's food is distinguished. She is an inspired, intuitive cook and it is I who encouraged her to write this book. I hope her readers will find it of value.' Political correctness is not a new phenomenon!

By now my parents had moved to Harrow in London and Nan came to live with us. She remained in close touch with friends, closest of whom were the personal staff who had surrounded both Sir Winston and Lady Churchill during and after the war. She also welcomed Lady Churchill's visits to our home. Once, in the early sixties, when Richard Burton had narrated the TV series *The Valiant Years*, based on Churchill, Lady Churchill rang Nan to say the actor had presented her with a colour television. Lady Churchill apparently already had two such televisions, so she wanted to bring it to Nan. Nan was delighted, but I remember her delaying the visit for a week or two as our house was the local Labour Party HQ for the imminent local election, and plastered in red VOTE LABOUR posters.

Nan was a great mentor and taught me to cook: main courses on a budget, starters that can be prepared hours or even days in advance, the multiple uses of cheap choux pastry, the benefits of concentrating on more labour-intensive but memorable puddings which work out so much cheaper. She supervised me often, always despairing at the mess that surrounded me. But then, I reflected, she did have kitchen maids to clear up after her and footmen to dish up. Much later she would come to my dinner parties and regale my fascinated friends with her stories – although she was always discreet. Now and again, after one or two sherries, she would talk about the day that Mr Churchill had asked to see the rations. She took them to him on a tray. 'Mmm,' he had said to her, 'not bad for a day.' 'Sir,' she replied, 'that's for a week.'

I started to trace the influences on Nan's cooking, and the recipes she chose to put into the book – as well as, more importantly, a few of those she did not include. Some favourites, such as suet puddings, were too simple or too cheap to be part of the collection. Others were perhaps too weird: on one visit to Bristol, she served us a fantastic orange pudding, which we were all demolishing up until the moment she told us that the main ingredient was potato. We instantly stopped eating and enjoying it. The published recipes also lacked Nan's vehemently held view that 'one never puts lettuce in a salade Niçoise', or the famous Irish stew that Churchill loved, and even the mousseline pudding. But just as Nan had learned so much from so many, she was clearly, as Lady Churchill put it, a brilliant teacher. Nan's enthusiasm for cooking and life in general, her kindness and energised commitment to a task shone through.

I remember cooking for her ninetieth birthday family dinner, a menu carefully planned with enthusiasm and precision. She drew pictures for me of how Poulet à la Stanley should be laid out and garnished on an oval plate.

By 1977, Mum was seriously ill with cancer and no longer so able to care for her mother. Nan was admitted to hospital with a chest infection and I visited her, to find her holding court with the doctors and nurses, cleaners and cooks. She was the only lucid woman on the geriatric ward and they were enthralled by her stories. She was released to a nearby care home, and Lady Churchill died shortly afterwards, on 12 December. I was with Nan a few days later when she opened her Christmas card from Lady Churchill – the handwriting is so frail. Nan's tears fell silently. She had lost one of her closest friends, and her daughter was terminally ill.

Mum died just a month later, and it was Nan who comforted me with warmth and understanding. I still have all the lovely letters she received daily from friends who had worked with her, expressing their sympathy for her double loss, linking Mum's death with the loss of Lady Churchill.

Aged ninety-seven, Nan died peacefully in her sleep, three months after Mum and four months after Lady Churchill. The letters I received from so many of her friends from those wartime years were moving, all recognising the value of their friendship as much as her cooking.

Some years later, in 1984, I saw pictures of the newly opened Churchill War Rooms and Churchill's bedroom. Beside the bed was a candlestick holder. I knew I had the original – Nan had always said it had been next to Churchill's bed throughout the war – a scruffy, cracked orange enamel candlestick holder. I rang the curator Phil Reed and arranged to return it to its rightful place. When the War Rooms were expanded in 2003 to include a kitchen I gave them more of my grandmother's equipment – the pastry cutters, knives, a waffle iron and a lovely carved tray, one of the many presents Winston Churchill had been given from the Commonwealth. I handed over those copper saucepans – and the links with her scullery maid's life in the kitchens in 1898, proudly maintaining 'the coppers'.

Nan was the ultimate example of active and healthy ageing, only relying on others for care in her last few months. She was independent, happy, fully in control of her speech and with a brilliant memory to the end.

It must have been so gratifying, at ninety-six years of age, to start recording one's life history with the following words:

'I feel I did give my whole life to the work I loved and enjoyed, and not only that but the most interesting people I served and liked who gave me the courage and inspired me to work hard and not to feel that I had no standing in life as a cook, but to feel on a par with other walks in life.'

2

It's never too late to find out what's important to you

Somehow a 'mistake' when I was ten led to my taking the 11+ a year early. I passed but being a year younger meant that I was hitting puberty later than the rest of my class and always struggling to catch up with my peer group. I remember my friend Helen wearing stockings to school ages before I was allowed to. I always had fat, mud-stained calves, and was acutely embarrassed by them. All my school friends were wearing stockings over their long slim legs and I was still in socks. I remember my mother ensuring I had sensible brown Clarks lace-ups, measured for size and width. I hated them, and once round the corner and out of sight from home I would take them off and put on a trendy, but ill-fitting, pair of slip-on shoes. The long-term damage to my feet is still visible, with my big toes forever distorted and my already wide feet never fitting easily into shoes.

Dad and his brother were keen cricketers, but I don't remember my mother having any sporting interests.

However, Nan was a very strong swimmer – one of those hardy souls who swam in the Serpentine on Christmas Day. In her autobiographical notes she described seeing another child nearly drown, which made her immediately resolve to learn to swim. I am pretty sure she told me she had swum around the Isle of Wight. I know she had been employed to do banquets and events at Cowes Week, but as it would have been a fifty-six-mile swim, I can't have remembered accurately – that is far too far. Maybe it was swimming across from the mainland to the Isle of Wight.

My all-girls convent, La Retraite, was not big on sport, and we had no access to athletics facilities. Hockey, tennis, netball and irregular coach trips to a swimming pool were all that was on offer. In netball, I was never tall enough to shoot or be a defender. So centre it had to be. But I loved it, and as my first experience of team play I recall my dogged determination and the strong commitment to the netball team of Our Ladies House, one of the seven houses in the school, across all age groups. That team spirit within Our Ladies meant I was always prepared to give it my all – perhaps this was the origin of my competitive spirit.

I was never the easiest of children to manage, and was probably viewed as rebellious and challenging. I remember my parents received a summons to come in to see the headmistress, Mother St Paul, when I was about fourteen. Expulsion was considered, but then an alternative was offered: it was suggested that I go to another La Retraite school, at Weston-super-Mare, where I would have to be a boarder. Fortunately, my parents couldn't afford the fees and I have no idea how Dad managed to ensure I remained at La Retraite in Bristol, but from all his writings and court work his thoughtful and persuasive skills were evident. By now he was Chair of the Juvenile Court and he once told me he was dreading the day that he would have to 'stand down' from the Bench because his daughter was brought before the court for delinquent or disruptive behaviour, or even being 'beyond control'.

I was never good at hockey. I used to be put on the wing, and never connected the stick with the ball very well – my hand–eye coordination is appalling. I still recall the embarrassment of having to go to school with that new hockey stick – a Christmas present from my father. It was one of the first curled-up new 'Asian-style' sticks. Embarrassed, and hating to feel different, I went to school with it at a time when all the other girls had the more conventional style. But yet again Dad was in the know and those sticks are now the norm. My best memory from playing hockey on Clifton Downs is of Peter O'Toole watching us when he was doing a season at Bristol Old Vic. Perhaps more accurately he was watching our hockey teacher, whom we all assumed he fancied.

As for tennis, I was absolutely useless – again, my lack of hand–eye coordination. Many years later I tried to teach my ten-year-old son how to take a backhand out of the back left corner of a squash court. I repeatedly hit the wall with my racquet, missing the ball completely. I watched in total astonishment as he roughly copied my action. Somehow he didn't hit the back wall, but picked up the ball and sent it down parallel to the side wall. Sickening.

I used to go with my father regularly to watch Bristol City play soccer, or to the County Ground to watch Gloucestershire play cricket. I loved the ambience, but in the fifties, sadly and frustratingly, those sports were not an option for girls.

Although not considered a formal sport, or recognised as 'physical activity', we would walk miles on a daily basis. La Retraite School was in Clifton, not far from the Suspension

Bridge, so we would walk two or three miles every day to the centre to get the bus to and from school. Added to this, as we played rounders or running games every break time we had good cardiovascular fitness. We would also play hopscotch over squares marked out with bits of stone, which must have added to our core stability and leg strength.

At home, I loved climbing trees in the local woods, playing ball games out in the street and tobogganing down the nearby slopes when the snow came. And above all, I loved roller-skating. Our house lay on the border between Somerset and Bristol and the pavements on the street outside the house reflected that division. The Somerset pavement was tarmacked. The Bristol side was uneven paving slabs, but a better surface for roller-skating and hopscotch. It is interesting to reflect on the significance of these play activities for crucial muscle and bone strength, and for balance. Will the youngsters of today not only be more obese, but also lack that early build-up of strength, given their sedentary, screen-based lifestyles?

When I was fifteen – and after getting surprisingly and unexpectedly good grades for my O levels – my family moved up from Bristol to live in Harrow. My father had been appointed Secretary for Training at the Association of Boys' Clubs, based at the Bedford Square headquarters in London. I went to the local co-ed grammar school in Edgware. There we had our own athletics track, but I was never any good as the rest of the school had been running for years, and anyway, after ten years in an all-girls convent I had other interests. There were boys in my new sixth form.

I also had my first paid jobs, either holidays or Saturdays, and I learned so much from those varied experiences. I worked behind the counter at Boots, then in the kitchen at Edgware General Hospital. After a brief period controlling the dishwasher, I moved up to helping the chefs – I have a vivid memory of preparing and taking up to the wards the 'final requests' from dying patients. One summer I worked cooking for students who were working on a strawberry farm, and regular Saturdays in a record shop in Harrow, when different recordings of the song 'Volare' were hitting the charts. I remember the record producer Mickie Most coming in to enquire how sales of his version were going.

My A-level results were nowhere near as promising as my O levels, and I barely scraped enough in maths and physics to take up my place at Nottingham University. There, I was still one of the youngest in my year, and aiming for an honours degree in maths.

Despite the facilities and opportunities, there was very little sport on offer at university that appealed to me. Early on, I went along to an athletics session and, after no warm-up, completed six brilliant long jumps. Maybe I had found a sport I could enjoy. But in those six jumps I destroyed my quads and could hardly move for the next three weeks, so that was the end of my membership of the University of Nottingham's Athletics Club. However, I did start ballroom dancing and really enjoyed that throughout my three years. I took medals each year: bronze in my first year, silver in my second year and finally a gold medal in the third year. Rather than dancing my medal tests with our instructor, I preferred to do them with my dance partner, John, a tall Nigerian athlete reading electrical engineering. Although the tango and foxtrot featured in our medal dancing, John had a great sense of rhythm and we both loved rock 'n' roll, the cha-cha and the twist. It was a highlight of my university sporting life, representing Nottingham University in the twist at a competition in Leeds. We chose to tackle it with John's more casual, minimalist approach in preference to the prevailing Chubby Checker energised style.

Apart from dancing, the major highlight of university was meeting my husband Phil when we were going to the freshers' parties of the first year. In the first few weeks I realised I was not interested in proving the existence of 1 and changed from maths to economics and psychology – something I was far more interested in (and maybe because the ratio of boys to girls reading economics at Nottingham in those days was 52:2). Phil was another first-year student, reading civil engineering. He had a long history of playing football and basketball at a good level. I now began my many, many years of standing on touchlines supporting him, and, later on, doing the same for our three offspring. I even supported the University relay team of which Phil was a part, pushing a pram overnight from London to Nottingham. Maybe this was the beginning of my dreams of one day doing something similar, for instance a long-distance relay like Race Across America. Both Phil and I loved our time at university, making long-lasting friendships and having a lot of fun.

In 1963, with my BSc in economics and two years of psychology almost under my belt, I briefly contemplated a career in marketing or even computing – I was in one of the first years to have the opportunity to integrate technology, and basic computer programming was part of our economics and statistics course. Adjacent to the economics library was a small room containing the *only* university computer. I recall reading *The Hidden Persuaders* and was aware that my economics, statistics and psychology, not to mention the very, very early days of computing had formed a degree that could equip me for a great entrepreneurial future. However, when I visited the careers advisory service I remember asking a somewhat surprised adviser how I could develop my long-standing ambition to be a cook like my grandmother. Rightly or wrongly, he was unequivocal: I would have to go right back to the beginning and train in cooking, and this might be a waste of my degree. My second option was more akin to my father's work in youth justice, optimising the chances of deprived young people.

Where might I have been without that paternal influence and my final decision to begin my fifty years of social work? Leaving university and still only twenty years old, I was deemed too young to go on a postgraduate social work training course. Instead I chose to get some invaluable experience in residential social work at a girls' hostel in Slough, run by London County Council. I learned so much from the young girls who came from complex family situations. Despite the long, long hours, I loved it. Following that I became a childcare officer, based at the Elephant and Castle — just up the Walworth Road from where some Silverfit sessions are now based. Unlike the affluence in the flats overlooking the Oval cricket ground today, back then the families living in those flats were struggling to survive.

I had to be able to use a pool car for my job. I had learned to drive when I was seventeen, as Phil's father was a driving instructor. Then a year later, with no more driving behind me than the fourteen hours before my official driving test, I had to do a test for LCC. Accompanied by the assessor, we picked up a pool car beneath County Hall and out I drove, into the madness of London traffic. He directed me up around the chaos of Hyde Park Corner and then Marble Arch, where I stalled. Amazingly, I was signed off as a safe driver, able to drive a pool car for the council.

Phil's university career was a little more disjointed. He and many of the civil engineering students were superb — arguably too superb — card players. Far too many hours were spent card playing and gambling. At the point where our relationship was in jeopardy, with the hours Phil spent playing brag, they all showed me how they had switched to playing bridge, again to a high standard. It took me a long, long time to realise that they were playing for money again. Although Phil and I went on to play bridge together socially I was never good, relying primarily on my social-work skills to guess what hands people were holding.

Phil and some of his friends failed their second-year exams and their university careers were brought to an end. He went to work for John Bloom, in the pioneering days of the direct selling of washing machines: John Bloom placed adverts in national papers, and when potential purchasers wrote in expressing their interest in the bargain prices, salesmen visited them at home. The relatively high earnings of the salesmen related to the 'conversions' of leads to sales. Strongly encouraged by me, Phil earned enough money to enable him to cease working for John Bloom and return to re-sit his second year, get his degree and finally to go into highway engineering.

We married in a lovely newly built Catholic church in Kenton before setting off, in our little sports car, on our honeymoon camping across Europe. On the second day we arrived in Luxembourg, pitched our tent and drove into the local village to shop for food and wine. I can still picture the scene, returning in a beautiful rural setting, the sun shining, as a car approached us. Relaxed and at ease, Phil veered off to the left as the other car veered to the right. At slow pace we collided and came to a halt in a potato field with one seriously damaged door. Names were swapped and for the rest of our honeymoon many observers, all the border officials and even the doormen at the Monte Carlo Casino commented, *Oh, la porte!* Subsequently, a very official letter arrived, in a language neither of us understood. We never went back to Luxembourg.

We moved back up to Nottinghamshire, for me to work as a childcare officer in the mining areas of Kirkby-in-Ashfield. With an exceptionally insightful boss, the Children's Officer of Nottinghamshire County Council, a visit was arranged for us social workers to go 'down pit'. Women were so, so rarely afforded that valuable opportunity. It was a memorable experience, going down the shaft and then walking and sometimes crawling down that long, long tunnel to the coal face. To see at first hand the working lives of those men, down there for more than eight-hour shifts, so very far from the deep shaft that could take them back up to the surface, was utterly extraordinary and was to have a powerful influence in my role as a social worker within the mining community. It gave me such insight into family dynamics and in particular, for my future work, in adoption and fostering, the psychological impact of male infertility within a macho environment.

Over the years I have worked across the social work piste: residential, out in the field, management of two adoption agencies, and expert witness work for the courts – always with childcare and child protection as the focus. At one point, when Stephen, my oldest child, was a few months old I successfully applied for a post as a housemother in a residential children's home for fifteen young people aged between three and fifteen years. Phil took an informal role as a volunteer housefather, whilst working for the local authority in Highways. I know and totally accept that such an appointment with a young child would not be possible now and yet I can reflect on the benefits that the presence of a little one within the unit gave to the other older children. The intense experience of residential care and the acute needs of those youngsters from such disadvantaged backgrounds has remained with me for ever.

That experience and those I have had as a social worker

have given me endless opportunities to appreciate how lucky I have been. They have given me an optimistic determination to make a difference, to help those for whom adversity had dealt a hard hand. But it wasn't easy. Always the butt of media criticism, you were damned if you removed children from home and damned if you didn't. Fostering or adoption for some of these troubled children is never without risk. My court experiences were tough, with a sense that the articulate lawyers were in their theatre, able to play any part, take any side, to challenge the views of a social worker speaking from the heart and caring deeply about the outcome. Despite this, I know that I helped to make a difference for many children and their families, and fought on their behalf. And those families gave me so much: a value system, respect, a thirst for knowledge and a strong, strong wish to ensure that we reach out to those less economically privileged.

At the age of twenty-five, and by now with two young sons, we moved to Welwyn Garden City, where I worked part time, helping to set up a new office in Hatfield and finally made my first sortie into sport. One morning, having coffee with local 'housewives', we were happily recalling how, ten years earlier, we had loved our netball. One of my neighbours thought she had heard of a league that we might be able to join. That was enough. We became the Housewives team from Panshanger. We had a short spell of coaching and we absolutely loved it. Two of our team were rapidly selected to play for Hertfordshire, and I too joined them in the lowlier county third team. Sadly, I only had the opportunity for a few games before we moved to London with Phil's job. With hindsight, what a fantastic team-building and community-building opportunity it proved to be – physical activity, combating the isolation of young mothers, developing our potential for leadership, and new friendship networks, all based on shared sport were invaluable ingredients in a recipe that I tried to replicate years later when I founded Silverfit.

Down in London, I played a couple of games for a similarly low Middlesex team. But with two young kids and part-time work, it was a long way to travel for games, although the matches were sometimes in beautiful hidden squares in central London. By then the rules were changing, the game so much more fluid as bouncing the ball was integrated. With a new home, and pregnant again, it was the end of my netball career. I have remained interested and wonder why, as one of the highest participation sports for women, netball has never been included in the Olympics, despite being recognised as a sport by the IOC. It is great that England Netball is now promoting walking netball – I may yet find my forte.

Following another job change, as Phil climbed up the local authority Highways and Transportation ladder, we moved up to Northamptonshire. Now with three young children and working again part time, back in social work and fostering and adoption, I started to look at classes I could do that would provide a crèche for Kate, our youngest. Unbelievably, looking back, there were only two options in Northampton: weekly afternoon discussion sessions on the women's movement, or morning sessions of badminton and squash at a local school. Here, the older kids looked after the little ones in the crèche. The sporting option won hands down, and although I struggled at badminton, I could at least hit the squash ball occasionally. Later I played for the Mereway squash team and as a family we joined the local Dallington Squash Club. That led to great sessions with friends and neighbours, and the essential recovery drinks afterwards. Sport became an integral part of our family life.

A few years later the five of us went on a family sports

summer holiday organised by Northamptonshire County Council, and based at a local college. Everyone stayed in the campus accommodation, meeting for meals, and we each got to choose two sports – one for mornings, the other for afternoons. All offered great facilities and instruction. Phil and I went for windsurfing and squash, Kate did horse riding, and Steve and Gary had their first attempts at taekwondo and badminton respectively. For both boys, their activities were to lead them on to greater things – Steve ultimately to second dan (black belt), in taekwondo and Gary to be a junior singles player for the GB badminton team. The immeasurable bonus of that sports camp for our family was that it was all local. We were able to return weeks or months later to Pitsford Reservoir to windsurf and go to the stables for Kate's riding. Gary's badminton instructor also happened to be the county junior coach and Steve's taekwondo instructor at the YMCA went on to be a national instructor. But, more importantly, what a fantastic model of inter-generational interaction and physical activity as each family member experienced different sports and venues. It was a brilliant idea that merits repetition in terms of family wellbeing, perhaps as partnerships between current leisure services and public health departments develop.

A focus in life on sporting opportunities and physical activity is great for kids. But the role of parents in such situations is often maligned. For me, it was never a case of being a pushy parent, rather more of being a reluctant chauffeur. I spent hours and hours driving kids to remote training venues and to competitions, sitting, waiting, and writing social work reports. Phil used to run the kids' football team, and although in those matches you certainly saw a few of those really pushy fathers, and even one priest, who was coaching one of the teams, on the touchline, possibly working out their own frustrations and failures through the kids, that was not typical of most of the parents or coaches I met. My pushiness was only evident in my determination that each one of my children could swim competently. I spent many hours holding them up in the water, ensuring they didn't drown or develop my fear. Having endless swimming lessons and taking all those graded competency tests was absolutely compulsory for my kids. My aim was to be able to sit poolside, reading the *Guardian*, rather than ever have to get into the water again.

As the kids grew, the demands of the family diminished and I got a little more time for myself. I'd been the chauffeur and spectator for my kids' sporting endeavours for long enough; it was time for me. Was it too late to start?

Nearing fifty, a number of things piqued my interest in running the Nottingham Half Marathon. Maybe it was the thought of running down memory lane. Along University Boulevard, almost past Florence Nightingale Hall, the peace of the music school where I did much of my studying for my finals, exciting memories of a year in Lenton Eaves, and the route back through Woolaton Park and past the Queen's Medical Centre we had watched being built, to the Trent Bridge Inn of my twenty-first birthday party. Or was it where I had been when Kennedy was assassinated? It had been a brilliant three years at Nottingham University, so if ever I was to do a half marathon, this would be the one. What a fun experience could lie ahead. And then, for someone who had made her own wedding dress in which Nottingham lace had featured prominently, there was the prize: a square piece of Nottingham lace in a frame. A wonderful race memento, still the best I have ever had.

Tim, a consultant rheumatologist friend, had encouraged me and his wife, Jane, to take up a load-bearing exercise such as running before we hit the menopause, thereby increasing our bone mineral density (BMD). With menopause, he told us, oestrogen levels drop, which leads to bone loss – for some of us, this bone loss is rapid and severe. The risk of bones breaking when falling is greater, and I also knew that women are many times more at risk of osteoporosis than men, so it is crucial to get the BMD level as high as possible pre-menopause.

Our friend Mike was going to do the Nottingham marathon and I went up to support him. Having watched him sail through the halfway point at Trent Bridge, looking great, I was moved by his total depletion and changed appearance when I saw him again, half a mile before the marathon ended. He was in the zone and oblivious to our cheering. He seemed to have lost so much weight and looked drawn and haggard. Miraculously, once over the finish line, he recovered within minutes. Having struggled forever with my own weight management I saw running as a possible solution. My mother and grandmother were both well over size 16 and I didn't want to go there.

After his race, Mike encouraged me in setting the goal of a half marathon, assuring me that 'anyone can do a half marathon, even if they have to walk most of the time'. He insisted that the first half of the full marathon route in Nottingham was the fun bit: it was the route around our old haunts, and missed out the second-half figure eight and that soul-destroying drag down the windy 2k regatta course at Holme Pierrepont!

So I went back home to Kislingbury village, about three miles outside the Northampton town boundary, and informed Phil I was contemplating running a half marathon in three months' time. Without a shadow of doubt he delivered the real decider for me: 'You could never run all the way to Northampton, let alone a half marathon.' I responded with that life-changing, utterly defining 'Oh yes I will!'

I had twelve weeks to train. I started the next day,

confidently running out of the house, but admittedly walk/ jogging as soon as I was out of Phil's sight. But it was a wonderful journey out of the village, down Sandy Lane and past the gravel excavations of the River Nene which were slowly filling with water. Beautiful big birds alongside newly formed lakes, birds I have never been able to name. But for me, it has always been about the ever-changing wild flowers, the trees, the smells, the wind and the rain and the peace. And perhaps the feeling of achievement, confidence and wellbeing at the end of a run. The endorphins released after that first twenty minutes contribute to the euphoria and the point where discomfort seems to ease and the joy of running takes over. I was always happy to be alone, in touch with nature, admiring the views, reflecting on life, thinking through solutions to problems and the social work reports I was working on.

With my new role as a fostering officer, life was still pretty busy and not without stress. I learned so much from those inspirational foster and adoptive carers, with whom deprived, chaotic, unhappy kids seemed to settle and make sense of their lives. The discovery of sexual abuse emerged in 1984. As we read more and more about historical abuse, I realise I was in the forefront of child protection in the seventies. Until then, physical abuse was the predominant form of child abuse. Like neglect or emotional abuse, sexual abuse had not been high on anyone's agenda. But then some of my former colleagues now working in the NSPCC went over to the States, learned far more about the identification and long-term consequences of sexual abuse, and came back to train us. The NSPCC skilfully fed the topic of child sexual abuse into tabloid headlines the day the inquiry into the death of Heidi Koseda was published – an inquiry in which the NSPCC was very strongly criticised because one of their staff had falsified their records. What a coincidence!

But without a doubt, we failed to protect some children. The choices we faced, however, were never easy and bringing a child with a troubled history into foster or adoptive care is never without risks. I look back on those days of the seventies and eighties and reflect on the indicators that we missed, our own ignorance of trafficking, of girls going missing from residential care, of abuse within families, residential environments of schools or churches, or within sporting activities.

By this point, sleep was in pretty short supply. As our kids became teenagers, the time of day at which I could relax and concentrate on report writing got later and later. But I seemed able to manage on five or six hours' sleep a night. I knew my grandmother had managed on even less, so maybe it was in the genes. But I had a goal. I was determined to complete the half marathon and prove my cynical husband wrong. After all, he was the sporty one – I was just the support team.

I was really lucky to be linked up with Chris, a health visitor friend of a friend, who also wanted to do the Nottingham half marathon and had done one before. In our twelve weeks of running together, she steered my training. But more than that, she took me out to the fantastic hills (well, maybe slopes) of Stowe and the flora of the woodlands of Everdon Stubbs. We put the social work and health visitor worlds to rights as we ran and chatted, steadily increasing the distances, maybe two or three times a week, sharing our experiences of the day, of the week, of life in general. Chris would wait patiently at the top of a hill for me to catch up. We varied routes, sometimes more urban, but mostly rural. It was an incredible and scenic introduction to the joys of running. Above all, running was the ultimate stress-reducer and energiser. I could go out, highly stressed, profoundly affected by the pain of some of the children and parents with whom I was working, and come back with their awful pain still there but somehow feeling stronger emotionally, more able to manage. Or I would go out feeling absolutely exhausted and return happier and energised.

The longest run I did was eight miles. I can still picture that summer evening. I was running alone and can visualise my total exhaustion at five miles, at a very specific rounda-bout, with three miles still to get home. How could I ever run 13.1 miles? What a feeling when I finished that training run. Is there a greater feeling of satisfaction than completion of a run – mission accomplished.

We were all signed up and the race numbers had arrived. Our neighbour and good friend Bob was also running the race and he took me up to Nottingham. No one in my family was particularly interested, or maybe free, to come too. Chris was a faster runner than me, so we had decided we would run our separate races and meet up at the end. Sadly, on the day, she had a raging toothache and struggled to get round. I was a bit surprised to catch her up at halfway and after that we ran together. For the first time I experienced the camaraderie and humour of the other runners, and the energising impact of the supporting crowds. We were all in it together, having fun.

The whole event was exciting, running through the throngs of Nottingham, past so many familiar sights before reaching Woolaton Park, which I know so well. A quick pop to a loo in the park and I was sitting down in sheer exhaus-tion, wondering if I could ever get off that comfortable seat and get going again. But after that essential rest, I was back on my feet and on to other familiar university sights: Lenton Eaves, the new hospital, the engineering blocks where some-one got their sums wrong and the two separate buildings were not quite the right height for the passage to connect them – we had thought this ironic for engineering blocks, and blamed its famous architect, Basil Spence. Then, in 1962, I had to have my tonsils removed in Nottingham Hospital and I ended up in the next bed to his wife and learned he was not to blame!

Finally, as we came back towards Trent Bridge, there was the division split – half marathoners to the left, full marathoners to the right. I remember noting how much fitter and healthier the half marathoners looked compared with the emaciated bodies of those running on. But I really felt for them. What did it feel like to only be halfway round? Never, ever, I told myself, would I put myself in their position.

The joy of collecting my first Nottingham lace trophy was incredible. I was so, so proud. Less joyful, though, was the experience five minutes later when my calf suddenly cramped as I walked back towards Bob's car, let alone the journey home, stiffening up by the minute. But what a great day and such huge satisfaction. An experience to be repeated. Could I make it round a bit faster than 2 hours, 16 minutes? It's all about personal goals for me, not about winning or beating another competitor.

By 1992, after seventeen years in Northamptonshire, the kids had left home and life was just settling down. Running was by now part of my life. Phil had risen to the top and been appointed County Surveyor, County Architect and County Planner of Nottinghamshire. We moved back to Nottinghamshire and our familiar university roots. We were overjoyed; it felt like returning home for both of us and I could continue my work as an independent social worker in Derbyshire and Northants. Always politically aware, like my dad, I would have loved to get into local politics, but we knew that Phil's senior role within the local authority effectively prohibited specific party allegiance for me.

One of the first things Phil learned in the new job was that

Nottinghamshire County Council was to host Velo-city the
following year. This was an annual international conference
organisation that moved around the world and had a wonderful mix of participants from the worlds of highway engineers,
cycling enthusiasts and politicians – or, in more formal terms,
was 'the ultimate platform for policy-makers, experts and
cycling advocates working for a world where more people
cycle more often and where the world's top experts in active
mobility, sustainable transport, city planning, industry and
cycling advocacy come together and exchange knowledge,
experiences and visions'.

Phil and a few of the councillors were scheduled to go
to the Montreal edition in 1992 to learn how Velo-city
was organised – the conference programme, the social life,
accommodation needs and, above all, the potential hire or
use of bikes. Raleigh in Nottingham were to be our UK
sponsors. Phil and I decided that I would self-fund and go
with the small group. I knew very little about cycling and
hadn't been on a bike since I was a kid, so I chose to attend
the vast range of lectures and seminars. I learned about cycle
path designs, about encouraging women in saris to ride, about
ways in which other countries' train and even bus systems
actually facilitated cycling, with attached trailers or bike
racks. Even now the provision for cycles on Britain's railways
is woefully inadequate, and certainly does little to promote
cycling or more active lifestyles. And, if we are going to age
more healthily, then far more focus is needed on safer cycling
lanes. I learned too that an early Road Research Laboratory
study had explored safe combinations of physical activity on
pathways, combining cyclist with walkers, or runners with
walkers. They found the former to be more flexible and
accommodating. Runners, it seemed, were often 'in the zone'
and less able to move to accommodate oncoming walkers.

Kids in helmets, I learned from recent research took more risks. They thought they were Superman.

A brilliant component of the four-day Velo-city conference was the opportunity to get out on bikes that the conference sponsors provided and ride through the local area. Our guides were fantastic, both in terms of encouraging our cycling skills and showing us the countryside and towns they loved. They were the cycling division of the Mounties, in their turquoise Lycra kit. When I asked what led such highly qualified, bi-lingual officers to choose to join the cycling division I understood research to have indicated that the kit featured in their motivation! What fun and what a privilege. I loved the experience and although I was rarely to get on a bike again for the next ten years, the attraction of the scenery and companionship stayed with me. Or maybe it was the vision of those Mounties in their turquoise Lycra.

3

Running to survive

Living in East Leake, I quickly got in touch with a small local running club, the South Notts Athletic Pacers. There were never more than fifteen of us, and for the most part fewer than that. I loved our runs. It is a reasonably undulating area so, for me, there were many silent uphills, while I let others do the talking. I did a couple more half marathons in Nottingham. They were a tiny bit faster, but never brilliant times. The intersection in West Bridgford, where the route splits before the second half of the marathon sets off around Holme Pierrepont, remained a vivid reminder of the insanity of running a full marathon and an effective barrier for me.

I had never heard of strength training in those days – the gym was all about the treadmill and a few chest presses. Now I realise I had found other ways of increasing my bone density and reducing my muscle loss as we carried out improvements and built extensions in several homes – I was an excellent labourer. When we had moved down to Northamptonshire, we both missed the Peak District and the opportunities for fabulous walks in such great countryside. I was self-employed and would have little access to a pension so, despite my political resistance to second-home ownership, we bought an old farmhouse, Blackclough, in the Peak District, effectively as my pension. We spent years working on its renovation. It was all hard physical labour, digging footings, mixing tons of concrete, re-laying floors by removing and then replacing huge stone slabs, and rebuilding the historic stone walls so typical of the area. It was therapeutic release from the pressures of our work and good strength training.

So when we moved to the Old Station House, our new home in Nottinghamshire, much renovation work was required. Phil was the engineer and craftsman boss, so again I was the builder's mate. Facing a few financial pressures, we hired tower scaffolding and it was my daughter Kate and I who painted the whole external face of the largish house, stretching up to the high pointed eaves. We even attempted, without total success, to lay tarmac on the drive. It was delivered to us in a huge hot pile, but cooled far quicker than we envisaged, hence a rather lumpy drive. That was embarrassing for the boss of Highways in Notts. But on reflection, it was perfect high-intensity effort and yet more strength training. Life was good: a lovely home in a great village with a strong community and even a local running club; Phil had reached the top of his professional tree; I was happy as a guardian *ad litem* (independent social worker) for children who were the subject of court proceedings; and the children had left home and were all thriving.

Cancer came so quickly. Phil's odd problems had been written off as stress related – his senior local authority post was certainly not without pressure. In hindsight, there was an indication in March 1994. Just before we went skiing with friends, I noticed that he seemed unusually exhausted on the cross-trainer. We were both a bit surprised; then in France he ducked out of a couple of long days' skiing, but nothing really significant. It was a great holiday and we came back to plan and construct our new conservatory. Maybe going off his food should have been another sign, but then he was always unappreciative of the healthy, high-fibre, high-protein offerings I dished up – rabbit food, as he described it. It was never as good as his mother's cooking, or his grandmother's apple pies.

Then suddenly, one night he had spasms of acute pain. It was Good Friday. Our doctor was called and Phil was rushed into hospital with suspected appendicitis. The next morning will be etched in my memory for ever. Phil was sleeping and I noticed the nurses didn't, or wouldn't, make eye contact with me, but suggested that we spoke to the doctor immediately. That young man was incredible as he explained the nature of the cancer to me and to Kate, who was by now a final-year medical student. We were both in a state of shock, and the skill with which he managed to impart information on such different levels was impressive, and I appreciated it.

Phil had surgery to remove a malignant growth in his colon. He took it all in his stride and left hospital shortly after. A few days later, armed with reports and X-rays, we all went back down to Northants to see the same doctor friend who had motivated me to start running. What a friend – someone who can sit down and go through the extent to which the cancer had spread, the risks, the prognosis. How important it is to know the odds, to face things together, to share.

Over the summer Phil recovered quickly – only now do I know that being fit before surgery and that physical activity afterwards can speed up recovery from surgery or other injuries. On 15 August 1994 we had a great thirtieth wedding anniversary party in our large garden, which was beginning to look good – the benefit of all my hard work. The garden of the Old Station House was adjacent and parallel to the disused railway line. The railway bank, with a range of wild flowers, was part of our back garden. It was hard landscaping, but a botanical and architectural heaven.

We had so many shared dreams for the future. All the kids had flown the nest, their careers resolved – well, almost. We had come home to Nottinghamshire together, in a lovely home, with a great village community. We were both happy with our work and we were close to the Peak District. Life was so good.

The day after our wedding anniversary we started to build the conservatory. As usual, I dug the foundations and mixed the concrete. Phil poured it in and levelled it with the superb accuracy one could only expect from a highway engineer. By October Phil had had another scan, but he had not had results before having to go off for a two-week work trip and a conference in Israel.

Within a couple of days of his return, Phil and I went to the hospital for the results of the scan. It was 21 November. He went in alone, and ten minutes later I was called in. Together he and the consultant told me there was good news and bad. The cancer had spread to Phil's pancreas and he had less than six months to live, but it would not be painful. In fact, he only had three weeks.

How does one cope with news like this in late November, surrounded by Christmas festivities? We had to tell everyone our awful news in the Christmas cards we were writing. I handed over all my social work cases to colleagues so we could grieve together as a family. When watching the news, Phil and I realised that it only had meaning for one of us. We had to be grateful for the rapid pension/ill-health settlement that enabled Phil to take instant retirement and gave some

cash where it mattered, to tell me one night where the stop-
cock and the fuse box were. But above all, with unbelievable
generosity, Phil gave me permission to enjoy life, to keep
running, to stay in social work and to do my best with and
for the kids. He was so proud of them. I had started my PhD
at Leicester University, where I had first gained my social
work qualification. I was looking at the adoption placements
of over a hundred children, from their perspective, and that
of their birth family and adoptive parents. Phil advised me, so
wisely, to continue with my research – to give me a longer-
term goal.

Are the final hours ever easy? Are they ever really peaceful?
Phil's were not, and I was left with a strong feeling that it
was deemed politically correct to die at home. We did have
a choice – Phil was admitted to hospital, where more tests
confirmed his all too rapid deterioration and the spread of the
cancer. I stayed with him overnight. Nurses both at home and
in the hospital did discuss the options with us, but there was
definitely a feeling from the nurses that home was the place to
die. One consultant did mutter that I might not find it easy at
home, but it was almost as though he was scared of being seen
to be putting pressure on us to stay in hospital. Bringing Phil
home from hospital from that overnight stay, the day before
he died, he was ever the highway engineer – critical of my
driving and my hopeless lane discipline.

I can still see him mounting the stairs for the last time.
Then that last awful, desolate, sleepless night: just the two
of us, alone, as Phil drifted in and out of consciousness, the
kids in their bedrooms. Finally, at 6 a.m. a nurse came, then
our GP, then a fantastic Anglican priest who dramatically
brought Phil peace and relaxation. At 1 p.m., after one final
big hug, it was over.

Later that evening, drained and sleep-deprived, I looked

at the bottle of medicine Phil had been given as a sleeping draft and suggested I might have a spoonful. My almost fully trained doctor daughter couldn't grab the morphine off me fast enough and pour it down the sink. 'No, Mum, I'll get you something else to help you sleep tonight.'

Fortunately, humour has always featured strongly in my life, and the lives of my children, along with optimism and the ability to see the funny side of situations. The undertaker arrived, sombre, head bowed – an actor accustomed to a very difficult role, asking awful questions that have to be answered all too quickly by vulnerable families at a grim time in their lives. When you think of the hours that go into planning a wedding, equally major decisions about dying, funerals, burials and cremation are made in such haste. Questions flowed in rapid succession about dates, times, what sort of coffin, what clothes would Phil wear, but the last one floored us. It was a tentative enquiry about the depth of the grave. We looked at each other questioningly until Gary said, 'Mum, he really wants to know if you are going in on top.' We roared with laughter, and as the guy left he thanked us for being one of the best families he had visited in such circumstances.

Even the funeral had its fun moments. Close to Christmas, on 22 December, the vicar of St Mary's had kindly delayed putting up the decorations in the church. Earlier I had helped to run St Francis Children's Society, the Catholic Diocesan adoption agency based in Northamptonshire. So it was great inter-faith collaboration that Fr Peter Wilson, my old boss and good friend, was there to take the service – someone I loved working with. He had such a progressive view of Catholicism. He taught me to see and appreciate the good in people and I always thought that, from a social work perspective, I taught him to be just a bit more cynical, albeit always compassionate. Pope Francis now fits so brilliantly for both of us into our Catholicism, at the centre of so many issues of today, from poverty to wealth, fairness and justice.

We didn't think of everything – one of my sons had no suit, so happily put his father's on. We never thought of the reaction of Phil's work colleagues at seeing a younger version of Phil in the same suit they had seen him wearing in the office less than two weeks earlier. My 'adopted' son Chris Hunt too arrived, a bit late, also needing to borrow suitable attire – but bearing his gold medal en route back from his success in the badminton at the Commonwealth Games. His mum had died around the time he was competing in the national Under-18 badminton championships, so Chris has always seen me as his adoptive mum. I was, and am, so proud of my 'adopted' son, who has played badminton for GB team in three Olympic Games.

We returned home after the burial. The conservatory, the footings for which I had dug in August, now had a roof, but was still unfinished. In the corner of the garden was the part-constructed fishpond we had designed and I was now left to finish off. Fortunately it was without water, but Chris falling into that space was memorable.

Towards the end of the funeral 'party', I left the house and went down alone to the graveyard next to the church. There were the gravediggers, filling in the soil over Phil's coffin, over a metre below. That, I knew, was the space for me. My faith held me in good stead: one day I would join him, but not yet. I knew I was the lucky one and I resolved to make the most of what life was to bring.

Christmas came and went in an amazingly relaxed and fun pink bubble – the first time Gary had been sent a work-related case of bubbly as a Christmas gift. The taste for that, like my running, has never left me. And there, outside our home, on Boxing Day were my running friends, from the South Notts

Pacers, marshalling for their annual Turkey Trot race. I joined them and cheered the stragglers on in their final miles. We were just a small club but organising the popular race was our way of giving back to an activity we had all gained so much from – another lesson learned.

What followed was another turning point in my sporting history. I had tried to book some counselling sessions in November, when I was told Phil had six months to live – knowing I would be carrying quite an emotional load. But the appointment didn't come through until a week or two after he had died. I had done two years' training in psychotherapy at the Tavistock Clinic, so counselling techniques were all too transparent to me. In our second session I could see my counsellor felt she had her eureka moment when I finally cried in front of her. That was enough for me – couldn't she understand that I cried alone, cried with my kids or cried silently when out with my running friends? Running with my friends, I decided, was better therapy for me.

So, that was the end of counselling and the beginning of more running. Running in a small group, you could distance yourself, tears flowing, or let someone else do the talking particularly when going up hills. As a social worker, I was good at posing the odd facilitating question, which would take a fellow runner friend at least five minutes to answer and therefore get me right up the hill without having to speak. We also had a lovely system, that one of the group would carry a whistle, and when it was blown the front runner had to go to the back – often me, a long way back. I owe them so much. That small running group of friends, our three kids and my Catholic faith were my survival.

Around this time, the club signed up to organise a Reebok Running Sisters group. This was a great idea. Reebok

supplied a ten-week training programme for a small group
of us to get beginners into running, with an end goal of a
5k race. It was hugely satisfying for everyone – with one or
two of the beginners rapidly overtaking me, and certainly
beating me in the Nottingham 5k Race for Life! It was a
valuable lesson in the feel-good factor that emerges from
volunteering. Seeing the participants' remarkable progress as
they walked four hundred yards, ran one hundred yards, and
moved through the weeks, going from walking to jogging
to running in such a short space of time. There was pleasure
too in racing as a new small beginners team from SNAP.
It's not just about winning. Some, like Diana, Steve, Wendy
and Anne, have remained friends over the years. Despite the
distances as we move around the country, we stay in touch.
What a lovely supportive group they were at such a time of
loss. There is a fundamental honesty about exercising in a
small group. With no face-to-face or eye contact, runners
are more open, arguably less defensive. When you are at your
limit there is no room for bullshit.

By now, my children were based in London. Remarkably,
they took me into their lives in a way I don't think would
have been the case if they had had two parents. Friends,
too, were brilliantly supportive. Before Phil's death we had
planned a ski holiday to the French Alps for the following
year, 1995. Tim and Jane and other friends and their families had been brilliantly supportive, giving me that strength
I needed, so I decided to stick to the original plans and go
with them. It proved a memorable experience, emotional but
nevertheless therapeutic.

After only three or four seasons, I was not a good skier –
red runs and a very occasional, cautious black run were my
limit. Then one evening we went up on the last lifts to the
glacier near Tignes. At the top, the sunset over the mountains

was absolutely fantastic. Emma Jane and I stood silently together, her support unspoken. The tears streamed down as I faced my own, and Phil's, loss. Life isn't fair.

Then together Emma Jane and I zigzagged our way down the moguls – she far more competently, but both of us laughing and loving every moment. And then my knee twisted and it hurt – just a bit. Did I imagine the snap in my knee? But more bruised emotionally, I got my ski back on and tried, unsuccessfully, to carry on.

I knew that calling the blood wagon to take me down on a stretcher at that late hour was not going to be popular, and that it would lead to delays for all the staff going home. Luckily, we were close to the top of the Grande Motte Funicular, so gingerly I descended to the top of the railway. Reluctantly, the last staff left on the mountain agreed to let me go down in the funicular with them and all the rubbish they had collected at the end of the day. I don't think I have ever had such a scary minute, holding on to the rail for grim death as the train descended at an incredible rate – no wonder they don't take passengers on the downward trip.

The following day, the medics at the resort decided it was a minor medial ligament injury. They bandaged me up and gave me a posh support brace, and I contentedly settled for a day or two of reading, coffee and *vin chaud* until we returned home. After all, I was the lucky one. I was alive. I'd had a medial injury on a previous ski trip and I told myself it would only take a few weeks to heal.

Once back home, it took a while and an insightful locum, a rugby-playing GP, to realise the injury might not be that simple after all. He sent me for an MRI scan in Leicester. There I learned that I now had a disrupted/broken anterior cruciate ligament (ACL). As I came away from the hospital with that news, the tears streamed. Instead of going home,

I made my way to the home of friends in the city. With this news, my real loss had suddenly hit home. I was on my own, coping with whatever crises life threw at me, small and large. After thirty years of marriage, this was the tough reality of widowhood.

I rested for a while and then started running again. I was reassured that half the England rugby team had no ACL. My daughter's research indicated that the population without ACL divided into three: those who needed immediate surgery; those whose knee kept giving way and would eventually need surgery; and those who for inexplicable reasons had good proprioception and for whom it appeared to make no difference. But I will never forget the words of the consultant: 'You will need to keep your quads, hamstrings and glutes strong for the rest of your life, or your knee will start to give way.' Less scientifically, but with a lot of experience and evidence, the medics in the ski resort the following year said they found that those with good muscle strength before an ACL injury (gained from running, or a similar load-bearing exercise) always seemed to fall within that lucky final group.

So, the running really had stood me in good stead, especially if my bone mineral density was good too. Also, suddenly and unexpectedly at fifty-two, I was post-menopausal. Menopause is not as openly discussed as other major life changes. But my periods ceased and I had been extremely fortunate in not having to endure the hot flushes and other symptoms that often accompany menopause. I returned to my medical friend, Tim, and asked if I could stop running now that I had been through the menopause. After all, it had been on his advice that my main goal of running was to get my bone and muscle strength up pre-menopause. But he insisted it was just as important now to keep going.

The South Notts Athletic Pacers continued to be

supportive, with regular runs ending in a bar at the local leisure centre, or running up a gravel path on a nearby hill to
watch the planes descend into East Midlands Airport. Mostly
we ran along the lanes near East and West Leake, with occasional evening visits to a neighbouring club who ran along
the River Trent from West Bridgford. There was a regular
safe run for the dark winter nights, too.

But I felt my roots lay in Northamptonshire, where we had
lived for seventeen years, so I finally decided to move back
down there. Just before I moved, South Notts Athletic Pacers
declared they were too small to be sustainable and decided to
close down. The last thing they did was to secure a club place
at the London Marathon, and they presented it to me. What
an opportunity. I moved back south with a determination
and a spring in my step. I was on my way to a new life of
marathon running, minus one ACL.

4

Exercising with others makes it easier

I moved back to Northamptonshire, to a lovely house, near great friends and good running terrain. I was working as an independent social worker, now in Oxfordshire and Northants, representing the most vulnerable children who were the subject of court proceedings. However, with my children living in or around London, I eventually decided to return there myself. I ended up within a mile of the early childhoods of both my parents: my dad in Stockwell and Vauxhall and my mum in Pimlico. Even more significantly, I had started my social work career in 1963 on the Walworth Road, off the Elephant and Castle. I was determined to make the most of such a vibrant city. Every week I resolved I would do something different: go for a walk, go to a show, visit a historic monument or go for a magical evening run along the Thames.

Having run the Catholic Adoption Agency for the Diocese of Northampton and East Anglia, I was now working part time as a freelance social work consultant with Parents for Children. PfC, as they were known, had a twenty-five-year history as an adoption agency, taking on pioneering work placing children with disabilities for adoption. We were finding families and showing the world that these children didn't have to spend their whole childhood in institutional care, that they could experience the love and security of family life. I had huge respect for the founders of the charity and their innovative work. I had profound respect too, despite my political views, for the generosity with which the *Daily Mail* and *Mail on Sunday* featured the children for whom we were finding homes whenever they had spare advertising space. Many, many successful family placements were born of those 'adverts'.

I joined my son and his wife-to-be for the wedding of his friend Harsh in Kathmandu where I met new friends and learned so much about Nepalese culture. I also got my first experience of solo travelling and a big adventure. I guess I had become more confident in my single role. I was welcoming the opportunities that life threw at me and I also knew I was reasonably fit – so trekking wouldn't be impossible.

As my son left to return to the UK after the wedding, I went alone, on my own two-day mini-expedition to the foothills of the Himalayas, travelling by train and then in an ancient taxi. It was fantastic, especially the late-night trek, alone in the bright moonlight with one guide. I loved the whole experience, the solitude, the time to reflect, the beauty, the history and the culture.

I resolved to come back, perhaps with a group of us. So with the links I had established, I organised a Nepali trek the following year. Arriving at Kathmandu, we went up past Lukla to Namche Bazaar – the gateway to the high Himalayan region and in the general direction of Everest Base Camp. One memorable morning one of the Sherpa guides woke me early. It was still dark. He took me a mile or two up the mountain track as dawn broke. Finally, around a corner and there was Everest – the tears streamed. It was a memorable trip with a great support team. We would be returning.

Having left my running group behind in Nottinghamshire, I had resorted to more lonely and isolated training in London – not really my style, but I had that valuable club place in the Flora London Marathon. I owed it to my friends from SNAP to do my best, albeit with no ACL in my right knee. I read *Runner's World* from cover to cover but my training plan was relatively haphazard: no training zones, not even a heart-rate monitor. But I did have the experiences of two sons who had done it, one knowing rather more about pacing after a 3 hours, 30 minutes finish. 'Mum,' Steve insisted, 'the long slow run really is long and slow. Forget your "go fast, go slow" long runs and get the speed session in at another time.'

My younger son, Gary, had run the London Marathon in 4 hours and 42 minutes. With hindsight, this was the beginning of having fun in sport together – in other words, inter-generational competitiveness. He had told me that he had taken it easy for the first twenty miles, arguably too easily for someone who in his badminton days had been very fit. But his moment of truth came when an old fat woman, as he described her, overtook him. Supercharged, as I was later to find is the case with so many alpha males, he speeded up, passed her and upped his pace right through to the end. He proudly framed his finishing picture, the 4:42 clearly displayed on the timing gantry above him. Now that was a real target for an ageing mother.

The London Marathon magazine dropping through the letterbox brought with it a crisis of confidence. Is it really for me? Had the postman or friends in neighbouring flats seen the magazine? Am I really going to be doing the London

Marathon? Panic, excitement, fear, isolation. The range of emotions hit me. I was cautioned not to deplete my body by running more than eighteen miles in training. I stretched it to twenty to get over that psychological barrier. You weigh up the psychological with the physiological. I always believe you know your own body and mind. I still remember the pain of that first twenty-mile training run – along the Thames towards Greenwich, down into that incredible Victorian tunnel across to the north bank and somehow weaving back along all the new Canary Wharf structures and endless building works. A marathon starts at twenty miles, they say. I knew the theory, but I couldn't imagine that I could ever run another step past the twenty miles I did that day. But the ACL-deficient knee was standing up remarkably well to the pressure. I felt no discomfort and it never gave way. I really seemed to be part of the lucky third of the population with that injury. So enjoy the experience, you are the lucky one, I told myself.

I explored nutrition but not seriously enough. Fortunately, just days before the marathon I found High5, and used their brilliantly prescriptive guidance notes for marathon runs, although my dentist, a former Olympian, urged caution about the steady intake of sugar. The training had gone well, with no serious injuries. I remember driving the car one day and almost by accident feeling my quads – they were as hard as rock. Were they really my quads? I had no idea I had been building up such hard muscles.

Saturday's registration for the London marathon is fun. You arrive to 'Chariots of Fire' belting out from speakers and a long row of desks manned by cheerful volunteers. As you exit, race number, timing chip and assorted paraphernalia in hand, the real panic and doubt set in. Everyone going back on the underground around me looked so fit and young. They'd been there, seen it and got several T-shirts to prove it. Get a good night's sleep on Friday night is the advice and assume that your sleep the night before the marathon may be a bit disrupted. Don't overdo the pasta. Eat your usual breakfast. It is just a normal day. Enjoy.

I was organised for the early start. My local No. 24 bus could take me straight from Pimlico to the train at Charing Cross. As I breakfasted on a boiled egg, brown toast and two cups of coffee as normal, I watched from my window as the 24 departed regularly, across the road, every few minutes. But by the time I left home, to my horror, the 24 bus that picked me up was 'on diversion', re-routed away from the marathon route and all the necessary road closures. The bus driver too seemed shocked and unprepared. The re-routing had clearly kicked in before he had anticipated, and he was forced south of the Thames, ending up amidst other congested and con-fused traffic. It was a long walk from the point where he finally agreed to let me off to Charing Cross.

It was much later than I had planned when I got on to an absolutely packed train bound for the start at Blackheath. I experienced for the first time that last-minute solidarity. We were all in it together, even if we might not get to the start line on time. There was one final stop at London Bridge before the train headed for Blackheath, but no room aboard for those poor runners waiting on the platform, their panic-stricken faces far worse than ours. And little space on the train to put on my timing chip, new technology I hadn't under-stood. There was no excuse – the chip was accompanied by a very clear diagram – but as is the practice of so many of us oldies, I had been confident a young person would show me what to do, and in what direction the chip should face.

In fact, I sat next to a young lad from Loughborough University who showed me how to put the chip on. He was doing a PhD on hitting 'the wall' of total depletion in hundred-metre sprints. That 'the wall' existed at all over such a short distance fascinated me. We chatted all the way about the variables he was measuring. In his research questionnaire he asked about sexual relations the night before, as well as diet and training. To my mind, he missed an essential measure: wellbeing, or happiness – how did you feel on a scale of 1 to 5 that morning? All the metrics he was using were objective and scientific, with a total absence of any of the emotional issues that I knew, from my very limited experience, could influence my times. Days feeling good always made my running more relaxed, confident and faster.

Our chat succeeded in calming my nerves, and finally I was walking with all the hordes up the hill to Blackheath Common, to that inevitable endless queue for loos. In 1996, women participants were still a minority but there were nevertheless longer queues for us. That first year's experience of London Marathon loos has stayed with me, forever ingrained. I have visited loos is areas of great poverty and not seen anything like those on Blackheath. Never, ever, I told myself, will I complain about any loo anywhere in the world after seeing and smelling that pile of shit mounded up and over the portaloos, spilling onto the floor and even out the cubicle door. Most competitors are anxious. Surely that is a predictable factor? But needs must and I had no choice but to ensure the heap grew ever higher. In subsequent years the loo situation did improve, marginally, but even at my last London Marathon in 2005 it was far from ideal.

As I was running with the club place from South Notts Pacers, I was on the 'blue start' for club members. Having given an estimated completion time you are allocated a pen (A–Z). While the first two pens seemed to move off quickly, it took ages before those of us with slower predicted times finally got over the start. It was a slow, slow shuffling first mile before the race opened and eased out and the fun began. We were on our way. Until, that is, the blue and red starts came together. The club runners from the blue start seemed so much more competitive, shoving and striding out. I had been advised to take it easy, to relax, to enjoy those first two miles, but it wasn't easy to pace oneself and back off from faster runners.

Then we were onto wider roads and I saw friends from Fostering Network, with their small instrumental band shouting 'Go Eddie!' My name was printed on my T-shirt in big letters. I discovered that the larger the name, the more vocal the support from the crowds. I aimed to make eye contact with everyone who cheered me on, and made brief gestures of thanks to the police and marshals. Support is a two-way process. I usually proffered high-fives to kids as I passed, unless there was a crowd of young lads whose raised hands looked as though they would knock me flying. I have never been in that driven zone where winning the race is all, and there is no room for interaction or enjoyment until the end. Here I was, actually at the London Marathon! This wasn't a race. I was going to enjoy it.

That first year was memorable for other reasons too. Around mile 6, a guy came alongside me. We chatted briefly, as you do, and he went on ahead. The previous year he had run the marathon in 3:01, so he was a man on a mission, to achieve sub three hours. Several miles later we came across each other again; he had waited for me and then ran at my pace: 'My name is Eddie too and I figure I get more support staying with you.' We talked most of the way round. I was fascinated. This other Eddie had worked in China for many years. 'Tell me,' I said, 'why did the Cultural Revolution fail?' Always my father's daughter, I had grown up admiring the

Mao concept, albeit with some limitations. Our discussion and reflections were a great distraction, for mile after mile after mile. I loved it – this was what a marathon was all about.

There is also the fun of overtaking younger male runners. All sizes and shapes, they see an older woman overtaking them as the ultimate incentive. Miraculously, they suddenly find that extra bit of energy and zoom past, sometimes to be overtaken yet again. My visualisation to ease the pain, relax or find emotional equanimity was that picture on my son's wall and the gantry reading 4:42. But I didn't really need to visualise, I was so enthralled by the magic of the streets of London, past the *Cutty Sark*, Millwall football signs, a branch of Tesco with a line of men peeing against the wall. 'You lucky things!' I called out to them. Minutes later they'd catch me up and more banter followed – those were the days before Paula Radcliffe liberated all women by crouching down on the road during the race.

Over Tower Bridge, that absolutely fantastic moment. The runners and the crowds are so deep that you can only just see glimpses of the river, although it was great to see Emma Jane shouting for me on the bridge. And then as you hit the other side you see the sign indicating you are very nearly halfway. Down the Highway and what excitement as the lead runners, preceded by the car with the electronic timing clock on top, approach on their way back up from the Isle of Dogs. I remember stopping to clap and cheer the leading guys, who were still in a tight pack. What fantastic athletes.

The dockland miles aren't easy. You go past so many runners on their way back who are at least seven miles ahead. It is a long stretch with fewer crowds and less exciting views; it feels endless. Drink stations offer such a welcome short break though it does become an obstacle course as you tread over the cups and jettisoned bottles of water. Finally back towards

Canary Wharf and the cheering crowds, and life begins again. Ironically, this is the route of the new Big Half Marathon, but how great to start at Tower Bridge and finish by going back across Tower Bridge and ending at the *Cutty Sark*.

The last four miles, the magic of the shouts of 'Oggi Oggi Oggi, Oi, Oi, Oi' as we descend into the Blackfriars underpass. No supporters in the tunnel. The only sound is the feet pounding the road. Then you resurface into the sunlight, Big Ben visible in the distance and the cheers of the crowds. Many runners were by now are walking at the side of the road. Wistfully smiling encouragement, we are all at our limit, but we are in it together. It is a great feeling. And at the 24 miles sign, I am on target to beat Gary's 4:42. I am euphoric.

What an unbelievable privilege is that last mile. Down and around Big Ben, and into Birdcage Walk, over that efficient chicane where volunteers skilfully move the tape from side to side to enable runners who have finished and are homeward bound to get across the road – the marathon route packed full of tired, slow runners. And then we are at the Victoria Memorial and Buckingham Palace and the endless final hundred metres. I chased the last fifty metres to make it before the next minute clocked up. I made it to the line in 4 hours, 12 minutes and 50 seconds. The most fantastic and exhilarating experience. And I had beaten my son.

Then the fatigue hits you. I had extreme doubts that I could mount that little sloping step to have my timing chip removed from my ankle. There was absolutely no way I could reach down to take it off myself, but there was yet another volunteer, waiting to help. Then the medal was put around my neck, another photographer and in a dazed euphoric state I was off to collect my labelled bag from the lorry that had, transported it safely from Blackheath. Incredible efficiency. I watched in amazement and admiration as other finishers devoured sandwiches and burgers, wondering how they could digest anything so quickly after the race.

An unexpected benefit of my special link with the nearby Churchill War Rooms was that I was able to go down there and use their shower after finishing. But not before Phil Reed, the curator, opened up the sliding glass doors of the display kitchen I had helped to develop, to take my photo, proudly wearing the Marathon medal. With Nan's copper pots and pans, pastry cutters, knives and the tray in the background, I reflected how proud she would have been of her fifty-three-year-old granddaughter. I wondered too what sense the visitors with their audio-tour telephones giving recorded descriptions of the kitchen were making of that strange sight through the window of Churchill's kitchen.

Finally, the moment I had been so eagerly waiting for: to the pub to meet my kids, so generous in their support, and that first glass of wine. What a wonderful feeling.

But, as I recovered, I realised how much I was missing the support of my Nottinghamshire running friends. I had appreciated just running alone along the Thames, the peace, the solitude, the time for reflection – but not every time. I resolved to join a club in London. One day on the South Bank, I came across a small group stretching after their run. I asked when they met, days and times. They were very welcoming, but suggested I looked them up in *Time Out*, and if I didn't think they were the right club for me, there was another one, also based near by. What a lovely way of telling me they were the Gay and Lesbian London Running Club, and that Serpentine Running Club was just up the road.

The following week, somewhat apprehensively, and knowing no one, I went along to my first Serpentine club run. Based at the Seymour Centre up the Edgware Road, they meet on a

Wednesday evening, go out for a range of distances and speed runs and then back for a shower and the pub. Back in 1996, there were six hundred members; now there are more than two thousand. It is a great club and relatively inexpensive. In 2002, a few of us started to generate a bit of interest in triathlon, and now it is a highly successful tri club too. The higher than usual churn factor, with members often only in London for few years, means there are Serpies or ex-Serpies all over the world. I have raced in Singapore, Italy, Australia and the USA, and there is always someone in the crowd shouting 'Go Serpie!'

I quickly met other Serpies, Grethe, Owen, Beate and Ron, living near me and our 7 a.m. Tuesday-morning runs before work became a regular feature of my week. Meeting in Pimlico, we'd jog to Battersea Park. Just the fact that one or other of us would almost certainly turn up at the meeting place was the incentive to get up on a cold, dark winter morning. When dawn coincided with our run, we'd see some of the Buddhist monks at the Peace Pagoda overlooking the Thames. On lighter spring mornings, the joy of running down an avenue of cherry blossom, the beautifully planted gardens, the Barbara Hepworth sculpture framing the lake, and that awesome 1k strip parallel to the river where we'd aim to do some higher-intensity sprints. I loved those Tuesday-morning runs, which were steady enough to chat, and enjoy the social element.

The Serpentine Running Club is a fantastic club, non-ageist, and welcoming to all standards. It is the rock on which I have built a social and sporting life. I took the opportunity to 'put something back' by volunteering and went on to help organise their social programme for a few years, and then act as the welfare officer. Amidst the bankers, journalists, accountants and lawyers, I was one of the few social workers. I also helped to organise the annual trip to Club La Santa in Lanzarote and a memorable Christmas Party down in the Churchill War Rooms when the emerging Churchill Museum was still a vast empty space that had housed the archives from The Treasury in Whitehall. The caterers even prepared a menu based on my grandmother's recipes and we gold-sprayed old trainers (that had been washed first) for the table decorations.

Best of all was our weekly Tower Bridge run, and the socialising that followed. Clive, a 2:38 London Marathon runner, would lead out a group of us every Wednesday night. That sense of magic has never left me; leaving Edgware Road, down to Hyde Park and Speakers' Corner, and then a gentle slope down towards Hyde Park Corner, through the underpasses and down to Buckingham Palace. Then on around Green Park to Big Ben, past the remaining office workers and the odd MP or celebrity leaving the House of Commons, or Portcullis House. A mad dash across the Embankment and we were on the best route imaginable, all the way along the Thames to Tower Bridge.

What a privilege. And, always, Clive bringing up the rear. No one was going to be left to run alone in his Tower Bridge run. There were several agreed stopping points where the faster runners would wait patiently for us to catch up. Across Tower Bridge, we were halfway, and now on the homeward leg. Past the new City Hall, past the Thameside restaurants I've always longed to frequent, past the Globe with one or two stopping off at the pub on a hot summer night. Then the Eye, reflecting how some of us had jeered as it failed to be hoisted up at the first attempt, but is now the iconic sight we have come to love. Then back up on to Westminster Bridge, Green Park, and past the Cabinet War Rooms.

On one such Wednesday-night run I had carried the

handwritten notes that my grandmother had prepared for her cookery book. I had told Phil Reed about the manuscript and he asked to use it in a new exhibition they were mounting. With absolutely no sense of its value, I carried it around on our ten-mile run and posted it through the door of the Cabinet War Rooms in a cheap brown envelope as I passed. Some time later they notified me of its value for insurance purposes. It was valued so highly that I asked if they had a zero wrong. It is still there in its glass case, on loan from me.

By now, minus the manuscript, we cross over the Mall and head up towards Buckingham Palace. And to that magic sight of the Palace at the end of the road, noting the presence of the Royal Standard if the Queen is in residence. Even at 8 p.m. there were always tourists around the Palace. We reflected that we were just out on our weekly run. Exhausted by now, but with the expertise of a speedy, knowledgeable runner, Clive was always advising us to 'see the run in small bites', 'picking off one mile at a time' and following his mantra of 'steady, steady, consistency of pace is all'.

Finally back in Hyde Park and only two hundred metres to go, and Clive would say, 'OK, now go for it.' Pulling out every spare iota of energy, we'd race up the slope to the finish line of Speakers' Corner, have a group hug and walk or jog back to the Seymour Centre. Every week, a 10.2-mile run – what valuable training, what fun, and as we met up later at the Windsor Castle Pub, it was time to reflect on what a great supportive group lay within Serpentine Running Club.

Our Wednesday nights were invaluable components of my marathon training. We were a disparate group, widely diverse in our professions, classes, gender and races, not to mention athletic ability. But our weekly Tower Bridge run bound us together. I may have been the slowest and the oldest, but I was accepted and encouraged. There were always interesting people to talk to. Running just has that bonding ingredient. I remember a girl joining our group one week – earphones in each ear. I just didn't get it, and even asked her, 'Why don't you run on your own? This is a social run.' It was this group that created the ten-marathon club, with awards at a local pub some time near Christmas. They conspired against me, refusing to acknowledge that my six half marathons constituted three whole marathons.

The monthly Serpentine Handicap is another brilliantly sociable fixture. After a couple of monthly runs as a 'scratch runner', members are then given a handicap time, based on an expected finishing time. With the anticipated slower runners starting off first, the idea is that everyone will finish at roughly the same time. It a great event, in the iconic and beautiful Hyde Park, always ending at the café for a coffee or even breakfast. There is an associated annual prize, the Tom Hogshead Trophy, for the person scoring the most points in the best of eight races throughout the year. Points are awarded based on two criteria: the position in which you finished, with the first person scoring twenty points; and, importantly, the success or otherwise of nearing or beating your own personal best for the course. One year, in 2002 to be precise, I realised in August that I was in contention for the trophy. I began to take it a bit more seriously, and September saw me go weekly to my favourite Dell Café in Hyde Park, with that brilliant view overlooking the Serpentine, to work on my PhD thesis and also fit in a training run. The staff would watch my bags as I ran once or twice around the Lido. I managed to get the winning points, just, and was very proud, subsequently, to house the trophy for the year.

Serpentine also organise the 'Last 5k of the Month' within Hyde Park – a race that is always oversubscribed. Usually Serpies marshal – only occasionally do we compete in the race. Years ago my son Gary and I entered the 5k. Patiently, I waited at several points so that he could catch me up. He was complaining of a bad knee, or hip, and then, with five metres to go, I turned back, hesitated, and he went storming past me to the finish line. Furious, I recounted my indignation to Manuel, a Serpie friend. 'What did you expect of your son?' was his response.

There are and were some other great Serpie training sessions too: at Battersea Park track, or hill work with Karen in Greenwich. It was at Battersea Park on Saturday mornings that I first came across Frank Horwill – and on a few occasions I was allowed to join his select group of athletes. What a privilege to work with them, those hill reps, the leapfrogging, the speed sessions. Frank was an inspiration to us all, despite his endless politically incorrect utterances as he motivated us to push ourselves just that bit more. 'Frank, you can't say that!' was my constant plea as the club welfare officer.

One shout from him will remain with me for ever: as I circled around the Battersea track I heard: 'Take that bloody smile off your face, woman. You are in a race.' Frank used to come as the run coach on the club camp to Lanzarote. And he was similarly unmanageable there. One year, as the camp organiser, I met Frank at Victoria Station and thought he was safely en route to Gatwick and Lanzarote. No such luck. He ended up in Brighton and missed his flight, but somehow talked his way on to a later flight, free of charge. He was such a motivational coach, and pioneering in so many ways. Frank founded the British Milers' Club, and he formulated the five-pace training theory, which is still widely used by middle-distance runners. Many athletes, such as Tim Hutchings, Seb Coe, Steve Ovett and Chrissie Wellington, credit him with their success. No wonder the great and good joined him on his seventieth birthday. I sat next to Seb Coe's dad. After many years of treatment, Frank died on 1 January 2012, aged eighty-four, supported by many of his friends and coachees. So many great athletes came to express their sadness and appreciation at his funeral.

Club La Santa in Lanzarote had been the Serpentine March club trip for more than twenty years. Around eighty of us would set off with Frank, and later, as triathlete numbers built up, we took swim and bike coaches too. The 'holiday' or, more accurately now, the 'training camp', is huge fun, a mixture of hardcore training and a great social life.

The Green Team – the coaches and support staff – at Club La Santa is made up primarily of keen athletes from all sporting disciplines. They are an inspiring and welcoming group, and the facilities are state of the art. You can do anything from windsurfing to golf, badminton to aerobics. Mountain biking and spin sessions are on offer, as well as great rides around the island – albeit with a hill in both directions! There is also the opportunity for an older person to fall asleep, snoring gently on the outdoor pitch in the sun, in a 'stretch and relax' class – to the amusement of my fellow Serpies. It all feels so sporty, a million miles from the bars and beaches over on the other side of the island. We have been over there training at the same time as Olympic champions in many sports, Team Sky cyclists, boxing champions. The great and the good.

In a fairly haphazard way, Frank, helped by another Serpie friend, Matthew, would organise a handicap mile at the end of the training week. It is great that the Frank Horwill Memorial Mile is now a regular feature of the annual Serpie camp. Our trip also used to coincide with London Marathon training week so I was thrilled to meet Mike Gratton, who runs a company called 2:09 Events – as 2 hours 9 minutes was the amazing time in which he had completed the London Marathon back in 1983. It is incredible how little marathon times have come down in all those years. Mike was a source of great encouragement to me, insisting that age was just a number and that I could still improve my marathon time.

Influenced by all these inspirational people, I began to structure my training more effectively, read avidly and built up those long slow runs steadily, confident in the value of our ten-miler in the bank every Wednesday. By 2001, I was all set for my second go at the London Marathon. This time as a Serpie, wearing the high-viz red and gold club colours, there was so much more support. It wasn't just the crowd of them at mile 17 on the Highway, but all along the route, and from runners overtaking me.

By now a familiar route, that second marathon was more relaxed and great fun – I was getting just that tiny bit faster, though nothing like as fast as Sue Lambert, Serpies' star older runner, who overtook me early on and finished in an amazing 3:39, aged over sixty (albeit almost half an hour slower than her personal best of 3:15 in 1995). I managed to creep in under the four-hour barrier at 3 hours 57 minutes. I was going in the right direction, but there was a way to go still, I told myself.

My time meant that I now came within the 'good for age' range, and could get a guaranteed place. It always felt sexually discriminatory in those early days, as to qualify for a 'good for age' place in the London Marathon, where ages are banded in five-year blocks, men of my age had to provide evidence of sub 3:45 time, whereas for a woman it was sub 4:30. I realise they were encouraging women to compete, but it did seem a greater ask for a sixty-plus man than for a similar-aged woman. However I was the beneficiary of this, and I totally supported any ways of getting more women into sport.

In 2003 I would reach the new age group of 60–64. I often wonder about the enthusiasm with which we 'athletes' celebrate getting older. I am sure there are very few within our ageing population who are quite so keen to reach the next age group.

In the spring of 2002 I had had the good fortune to go out to Nepal again, trekking up towards the Annapurna region. We had timed our trip to coincide with the rhododendrons in full bloom, the purples, reds and whites. A fantastic sight. There, in a lodge, I celebrated my sixtieth birthday. Amazingly, our Sherpa friends had carted some bubbly and white wine up there for the party. We were joined by some of the Nepalese team who were hoping to be the first all-female team to do the Everest ascent. We donated generously to their mission.

Interestingly, we also met a group of German medics who were en route to the summit of Everest. We had been out there for three weeks and were on our way home when one of the doctors gave me advice about my forthcoming London Marathon, some three weeks later. 'Resist the temptation to do a long-distance run when you get back to UK. Don't underestimate the impact on the body of an aeroplane flight. If you want to make the most of the altitude training you have been doing, take it steady until the Marathon.' This was brilliant, firm and authoritative advice for an older woman who had been about to get back to London and calm her anxiety by undertaking a last twenty-mile run.

Lining up for that third marathon, with my 'good for age' place, was so much easier. The smaller green start was for 'good for agers' and also the celebrities, and those dressing in elaborate costumes. The atmosphere seemed far more relaxed. Frank Bruno alongside me, charming, wishing me well. No evidence of any anxiety there. But then, just as we waited for the start, we had a minute's silence for the death of the Queen

Mother. Heads bowed, we were suddenly aware that a guy just in front was having a pee. Laughter at the wrong time.

So, off we set, the most relaxed group I had ever started with. The super age-groupers were able to charge off, without the dense crowds of runners, to get into a good pace. The rest of us – oldies, celebs and the odd rhino – could move at our own steady pace. Then at about mile 4, we hit the Blue start runners. What chaos, and what anger those aggressive runners showed towards me and the other slower oldies as they passed us. They clearly hadn't appreciated, as our race numbers and start colours were on our fronts, that we had been on a different start. As they barged through in a congested road, they clearly thought I had lied on my entry form and, far too optimistically, placed myself in a pen with an upgraded time. The jostling and crowding continued, until the meeting with the red-start runners and finally the whole route widened.

In 2003 I found myself lining up yet again. It was another 'good for age' green start and all was going well. With target times written on my wrist, I was doing well. I find it fascinating how quickly I lose all ability to do any calculations after less than twenty minutes' running. Yet I can construct social work reports in extremely creative, insightful ways the whole way round. So this year, at every mile-post I marvelled at my improved times. Was I really on target for 3:40? Suddenly, at mile 15, I was running very close to the kerb when I took my eyes off the road and fell, my rib and front tooth hitting the top corner of the high kerb. I was down for a while before I saw the blood pouring from my mouth and realised I no longer had a front tooth.

The spectators and I searched for some while before we found my tooth amidst the debris in the gutter. None of us had any idea just how long a tooth plus its root is. I can now authoritatively say it is at least two centimetres. Just ahead, on a roundabout, was a first aid caravan. If you are going to knock a tooth out, do it next to the first aid station. They washed my tooth and put it into one of their plastic gloves. Disbelieving and astonished that I wanted to continue, they didn't stop me running on. My red and gold Serpie shirt was covered with blood but it wasn't too visible. My rib was distinctly uncomfortable, but I was still on an endorphin high so I joined the runners again, setting off towards the Mall with eleven miles to go.

Maybe it was psychological, maybe it was for real, but I found it hard to get back into the same pace. I debated silently on the loss of blood, and whether I should or should not continue. And then, from behind, came Paul, a fellow Serpie. He was a sub three-hour runner who hadn't been too well at an earlier stage in the race, but he was making up for lost time and was about to overtake me. In a wonderful and typically supportive Serpie fashion, as he saw my state he immediately slowed down and said he would stay with me for the rest of the Marathon. He did, and I remain eternally grateful for his care and patient, encouraging support.

Then, on Narrow Street, mile 16, there were my three kids; Steve with a banana held out as had been planned. I will never forget the horrified look on their faces as they saw the damage: blood still over my face and a tooth missing. Kate took the tooth off me and promised, as a good paediatrician would, to get it into some milk. Essential for a child's tooth, though less use for a sixty-year-old one, where it is more important to put the tooth back in as quickly as possible. 'Stop talking, Mum, you are in a race,' they insisted, so I went onwards, past the crowd of Serpies at mile 17 and back to the Embankment and those iconic views of London.

That final glorious mile, with no awareness of pain from

tooth or rib, I realised what fantastic anaesthetics those chemicals released by endurance running can be. Around the Victoria Memorial, and as we approached the finish, my time suddenly came into view. I was so, so close to going over four hours again. With an incredibly determined final push I was under the gantry, with Paul, in 3:59.29. Not bad after the delays and incidents. And then into the volunteers' support area. And there, in his pristine white volunteer's boiler suit, was my former next-door neighbour, Bob, who had done that very first Nottingham half marathon with me. I declined the proffered first aid, and after a hasty clean-up it was on, at last, to the Petty France pub and the kids, where my tooth was steeped in milk, or was it wine?

Kate found the number of the on-call dental service. After at least two (or possibly three) glasses of wine we were on our way there by taxi. 'We wondered if we'd get anyone from the marathon today,' said the staff at the NHS dental hospital. I received brilliant treatment and within half an hour they had my tooth in front of me on a table, giving it root-canal surgery. What a weird feeling, hearing the familiar sound of the drill as they performed the same treatment I had experienced several times. I am sure I felt the pain as they did it! Then back in went the tooth, with a brace to keep it in place. They assured me that it might last a year or so, and then would go black and have to be replaced. More than ten years later it is still there, albeit a little bit grey. And the rib? That was far less visible, but more painful once the endorphins and alcohol wore off.

By 2005, I was managing Parents for Children. I loved the London Marathon and thought it would be great to get some charity paces for PfC. I spoke with an organiser on the phone, and asked about the massive price that the London Marathon charge charities. If I, as an individual, could get a place for £22.50, I asked, why should Parents for Children have to pay £300 for a gold bond guaranteed-entry place? 'It's win-win,' he calmly assured me. 'You make money, so do we.' 'No,' I said. 'You are exploiting charities.' Bang went the phone.

I suspected that many purchasers of charity places did not know this pricing differential. I did try to raise awareness but, for the media, the London Marathon is a good news story, and other charities were not prepared to rock the boat for fear of losing the valuable income from their gold bond places. The Channel 4 programme *Dispatches* did finally raise the issue in 2010, but to a mixed response. But that year Parents for Children were fortunate to be offered some corporate-funded relay places in the London Triathlon. Then, in one of the teams, I only had to undertake the 10k run, but it was a fantastic introduction to the world of triathlon.

For my fifth and final marathon in April 2005, I was really taking it seriously – maybe too seriously. Initially it was all going well. For the first time I had stuck to a training schedule. I had done a 5k, from which my projected finish time was calculated. My 5k time suggested I could achieve a 3:35 marathon if I maintained the correct pace. I set off at that pre-ordained pace, but with hindsight it was too fast and by mile 10 the realisation that I had over-cooked it dawned. I slowed up a bit, and failed to meet any of the split times written on my arm. I finished in 3 hours, 45 minutes. Not the time for which I had aimed and trained, but nevertheless a personal best. A few weeks later a package arrived out of the blue – a lovely trophy indicating I was the second-fastest female in my age group. I'd had no idea.

But I was beginning to realise that I might be getting too old to push those vulnerable knees to the demands of a marathon. I resolved to focus more on multi-sport, and the shorter triathlons and duathlons I had begun to attempt a few years earlier. Never could I have dreamt that twelve years later I would walk/jog/run that same marathon distance after a 3.8k swim and a 180k bike ride in an Ironman triathlon.

5

Find your niche and the world is your oyster

I had supported my son Steve doing the London Triathlon at least twice. As one of the largest triathlons in the world, it always has a great atmosphere. Whilst on the sideline watching Steve in 2000, I suddenly saw Simon Lessing being interviewed. He was just back from the Sydney Olympics where triathlon had been put on the map. Having been world champion for several years, Simon had been expected to get gold. He had failed, finishing ninth. Whilst many athletes who had finished competing, including my 'adopted son' Chris, who had played in the badminton mixed and men's doubles, were still having a great time in the Olympic Village, Simon had come back to the UK and competed in (and won) the London Triathlon. I admired his resilience.

Watching Steve in 1999 and 2000 was the real inspiration, though. I knew all too well that I couldn't pound the streets for much longer, and triathlon offered a far more effective option to stay fit, and have fun. I had been to see a physiotherapist with a minor muscle problem – for which the solution appeared to be stretches and NO MORE HIGH HEELS! He had told me that a significant proportion of their business came from runners – not triathletes, who, if injured, could turn to training in the other disciplines. Encouraged by Steve, I was beginning to seriously contemplate doing a triathlon. I was worried, though, about fitting in the hours necessary to train in three separate disciplines – as I later found out, I was not alone in this. Still, in 2000 I resolved to do my first London Triathlon as an individual, rather than doing the bike or run leg in a relay team for Parents for Children.

The rest of my life was challenging and not stress-free. I was working full time as in independent social worker on complex childcare cases for the courts, and partly for Parents for Children. We were establishing a new project working with children whose brains had been permanently and pro-foundly affected by alcohol *in utero*. As is my wont, I had thrown myself into this major issue for society. This meant taking on the power of the drinks industry and the prevailing binge-drinking culture.

We had organised some fundraising triathlon relay teams for Parents for Children, and I even did the odd run or bike – but never the swim. It was a great way of raising funds – especially when the run route took you past the pub where the rest of the teams would support vociferously. But yet again, I couldn't quite understand why a corporate team should be able to get relay-team entries more cheaply than the charity could. A small tent for the charity along the route would have set Parents for Children back hundreds. The pub that was free access was a far better option! Thanks to the generosity of a great corporate firm, who paid for the charity places, we managed the process well with funded relay teams.

One year, Annie Emmerson, Tom Lowe and Phil Sykes raced for PfC and we were so proud that they won the relay competition – though maybe it was not so surprising given their combined skills as national-level athletes. It was a privilege to see how much these professionals had gained from sport, and triathlon in particular.

Perhaps it was the motivation and determination of these professionals that finally influenced me to have a go at a whole triathlon, knowing that the knees didn't need another London Marathon. But there was a major problem for this fifty-seven-year-old if she was serious about doing a triathlon: she could barely swim. I come from the generation and school where we only did about one term of swimming lessons at school. We were taken by coach to a local pool, where someone taught us to do breaststroke. Our heads always had to stay clearly above the water level as you didn't dare get your hair wet. There were no hairdryers in the changing rooms in those days, and the prevailing belief was that you'd catch a chill with wet hair. My fear of water wasn't helped by a nasty experience when on holiday in Cornwall as a child, when I was standing on rocks looking into the rock pool. Suddenly a big wave pushed me off the rocks. Fortunately the water below was not too deep, but I can still remember the experience vividly. So, all things considered, I was no water baby.

Having decided to have a go at learning to swim crawl, I went for a whole term of lessons at the local sports centre and still totally failed to master any buoyancy, breathing pattern or leg kick. The following term, I signed up again, but also went weekly to the shallower training pool and practised, confidently within my depth. It was there that I met Stephanie, who was later to train as a swim coach, and two other older women. In the December we celebrated our regular swims with mince pies – yet further proof that it was the social element that kept me attending. I worked so hard to relax and improve my uncoordinated swim stroke, and I was finally able to swim a whole length in the 'big pool', but oh, so slowly. Not much has changed, and I realise what a huge advantage it is to have learned to swim competently as a child: not just the technique and the body position, but the feeling of being relaxed in the water.

By now we had a tiny group within Serpentine Running Club who were also thinking of triathlon, and we even sourced some tri-suits. I bought my first, very basic road bike, a yellow Giant. That bike, having progressed to do duty as my grandson's first bike, has now been returned to my turbo trainer. I remembered a bit of bike-riding as a child, and found I could still balance, and mount it with that childish scoot and leg over. But real road cycling was a totally different thing. Was I too old? All the others in the Serpentine group were the age of my own kids. Had I left it too late? I vividly recall the very first time I climbed Box Hill with another Serpie, Quinton, in the old days when the road surface wasn't such a joy to ride. It later became the Olympic route and the surface is now so smooth – another legacy of 2012 – but in those days there were potholes everywhere. I was not used to road cycling, and was really struggling on the steep ascent. I recall the embarrassment of having to walk my new Giant bike up that final bend of the Box Hill zig-zag. The café at the top is my favourite, though, and their flapjack remains my ultimate goal for training in the Surrey Hills, despite the hundreds of cyclists up there now by 9 a.m. every Sunday.

My very first triathlon was at Crystal Palace in 2001. It was a sprint triathlon, and my first swim in a 50-metre pool – eight lengths felt daunting. This was to be followed by a 20k bike ride, and a rather hilly 5k run. I was overawed at the thought of entering the National Sports Centre, that acclaimed venue which had witnessed James Hunt driving, Zola Budd running, Crystal Palace football games, and was home to the famous cricket pitch where W. G. Grace was caught out by Sir Arthur Conan Doyle. So I went alone, anonymously, and didn't tell anyone. I was so scared. I have no recollection of a finish time; I just aimed to survive. Yet for the first time I experienced the euphoria of getting out of the swim and on to the bike, unsure which contributed most to my joy. The biggest challenge proved to be counting the nine bike laps accurately. The best part, without doubt, was the two-lap run in that lovely park.

Overall, I absolutely loved my first triathlon, and the combination of the swim, bike and run, within the beauty of Crystal Palace Park. I loved the fun with other competitors, the enthusiasm and support of the volunteer marshals and, at fifty-seven years old, the experience of being the oldest woman competing in the race and the thrill of that final sprint before coming over the finish line. Being the oldest woman in events has followed me over time, but it is great to see now how many more women are taking part, especially the over-fifties and over-sixties.

My next triathlon was at Hampton Pool – a fantastic outdoor pool, heated throughout the whole year. It is a weird but satisfying experience getting into that warm water from the cold outside, swimming up and down the lanes, under the lane ropes and emerging at the far end into transition and off onto the bike ride. The run was usually in neighbouring Bushy Park, but it was closed during the foot-and-mouth crisis of 2001, so there was an alternative run route. I didn't realise the beauty we had missed within Bushy Park until years later, when Parkrun started there. But I was really getting into the triathlon mode – even if I was always the last person out of the water. I was beginning to enjoy the cycling too, seeing the views and countryside at a faster pace than running: the quiet, the rhythm and often the solitude. I love riding alone, but appreciate that I don't push myself as hard and as long as I would riding in a group.

I was again organising the Club La Santa trip, and that year I realised we had a few budding triathletes amongst the Serpentine group going over in March. We had space to take a triathlon coach, so I rang British Triathlon and explained that there were a few of us, maybe fifteen to twenty, who were interested in cycling too, but that the range of competence was very wide, from some really good cyclists down to me as a total, very slow novice. They suggested Brian Welsh from Just Sweat No Tears as a coach who could cater to that wide range of ability.

I will never forget that first morning. Brian and I went at around 10 a.m. to meet up with what we had anticipated to be just a few fellow cyclists, only to find at least forty or fifty Serpentine Running Club members there, all ready and waiting. Although still primarily runners, they clearly had other skills of which we had been unaware, and had hired bikes.

We went on to have a great week on the beautiful volcanic island, at the resort that I love. A massive volcanic eruption in the 1730s led to lava destroying villages and covering much of the island. This gives Lanzarote a unique, unspoilt and wild beauty. The legacy of César Manrique still dominates. He was an artist and architect who masterminded the sympathetic development of the island and its tourist industry, with whitewashed architecture and the lack of tall buildings to blight the vista. The wind, as we have all come to accept, is part of Lanzarote – either bad or awful, but rarely non-existent. The road surface in those days was very bad, endless bumpy tarmac with holes, and scary descents when a spill meant being dumped into a lava field.

By now I could swim – just. I remember the day I privately set myself a test distance and finally managed sixteen lengths of the 50-metre pool. Although totally exhausted, it was a day for celebration. I felt confident enough to enter the London Triathlon as an individual for the first time, rather than as part of a relay team – back then, triathlons didn't fill up within hours of opening, so I was able to make this last-minute decision. I look back and think I was mad. I started to avidly read *220 Triathlon* magazine, and various books, and built up distances slowly on the bike and in the pool. The running was never a problem, an opportunity to make up time over better swimmers and bikers. The nerves were building up as August approached – the swim, as ever, the deepest fear.

By the Saturday afternoon of the London Triathlon, I was on my way to ExCeL to rack my bike – in those days they let you on the DLR with a bike. For the first time I had to manage the complexity of triathlon logistics, remember all my gear, not to mention a bike in reasonable working order, have the right clothes laid out, my hydration and nutrition sorted. I have never been the most organised of individuals, with a tendency to cram too much in to life, often forgetting essentials, so ensuring my race belt had my number attached, drink bottles and energy gels were in the right place, and bike and run shoes at the ready was, and remains, a challenge for me. Trying to remember exactly where my bike is can often be a challenge too, with row upon row of bikes racked on rails. I often claim my old age as justification!

However, with the bike safely racked, I went out for a drink with a friend to a riverside pub, to calm the nerves. Together we surveyed the River Thames, and wondered if I would ever have the courage to get into the water the next morning. Surely, I reassured myself, the water in the dock would be a bit calmer than the river. But was it deeper, I asked myself. I was desperately scared and faced a sleepless night. Morning came, and I was back on the DLR en route to ExCeL. Thereafter the camaraderie helped enormously. It wasn't just going to be me out in that water. Anyway, I had been told in the briefing how to put a hand up so that a canoeist would come to my rescue. And a wetsuit does make you more buoyant.

Ironically, at the door of ExCeL I bumped into some old friends I had not seen for years. They were there to support their son and, knowing of my non-sporty history, were utterly amazed to hear that I wasn't there on a similar mission. I was actually going to compete.

It was time to struggle into the wetsuit, hat on, goggles on, scary. The starts of over a hundred swimmers are organised into timed waves. You jump off a smallish pontoon into the depths below, hopefully surface, and then swim twenty metres or so to the starting point between two boats. Whilst others confidently jumped in on either side of me, I sat on the edge of the pontoon scared beyond belief, questioning whether I could even swim out to the start.

Finally, I was in the water. The klaxon went before I reached the others treading water at the start and I was off. I stayed right at the back of my all-women's wave. I swam front crawl for about two hundred metres and then did breaststroke for a bit. There were so many friendly canoeists on the water, and I chatted to several of them as I caught my breath – about the weather, the views, the bike leg to come, all sorts. Then suddenly massive turbulence, a blast of black rubber shooting past – the next wave had caught me up and were swimming over the top of me, underneath and round each side. Didn't they realise how scared I was? But then the pressure of that overtaking mania subsided and I was back to my calmer, leisurely swim at the back again. Planes were landing close by too, at City Airport — it was the smell of the jet fuel rather than the taste of the water that I noticed the most.

Watching from the far side of the dock, my kids said I was unmistakable, even in the distance, with my slow arm lift, and every few strokes a big kick with my left leg. But my sighting wasn't too bad — the buoys in the distance were clearly visible and I had mastered six strokes then lifting my head to ensure I was still going in the right direction. The last four hundred metres are alongside the ExCeL building, so every sixth strokes offered an opportunity to see cheering crowds — even my kids. It is amazing what a difference that crowd encouragement makes.

Exhausted, I finished the 1500-metre swim and needed all three of the helpers at the exit to haul me out of the water and pull me up the ramp, and perhaps even help get my wetsuit off and placed in a big polythene bag. With wetsuit in bag, you then have to mount the slippery staircase up into the main ExCeL hall. If I, with limited swimming background, and at the age of nearly sixty, can experience the joy of the transition from swim to bike, then surely anyone can?

The bike route that year was the best ever, just another bonus on top of the euphoric feeling of being out of the water and on the bike. It was an incredible privilege to cycle on closed roads, around the Tower of London, along the Embankment and through the all too familiar Blackfriars underpass of the London Marathon route — but no oggi, oggi, oggi this time. Then the ecstasy — along the Thames, to the turning point just before Big Ben. There was plenty of warning that there was a U-turn ahead, but no preparation for the fact that there would be an event photographer lying prone on the ground — he was trying to get a picture of each cyclist with Big Ben in the background. As I swerved to avoid him, I nearly fell on top of him. But it seemed like a high risk worth taking for such unique photos.

With so many different waves out on the course at the same time, there is little sense of where you are in the field. Most bikes passed me, including a friend, Ralph, with his shopping basket on the front – but then he was working as a bike courier at the time. At least I was able to count my laps. I think it was the following year my son managed his third lap in an impressive two minutes – strangely the techies didn't spot that incredible lap time, and his total time remained as that remarkable two minutes. Counting laps is challenging – even placing strips of tape on the handlebar leads to wondering if I had taken the tape off at the beginning or the end of that previous lap.

I was vaguely aware that my three supportive and enthusiastic kids were drinking steadily. As I completed the bike laps and then jogged up the slope to transition in the ExCeL building, the commentator Ian Pettitt seemed to know more and more about this older woman: social worker, first triathlon, awful swimmer. Ian never forgot that information and he was the first person I saw, microphone in hand, as I climbed, trembling, into the freezing waters of Llanberis to do my first ever Half Ironman. There he was again, telling anyone who was prepared to listen all about me just before we took the plunge. Later, as I came in on the run to Conwy Castle, there were his sonorous tones again, telling half of Wales about my life, my kids, my preferences in wine etc. But it has all helped lead to increased support and recognition for the 'older woman'.

The exhilaration of the finish of that first London Tri was something I had never experienced before in running. I had actually finished it – the kids assured me that their dad would have been absolutely amazed, and just a bit proud of me. Suddenly, I heard my name over the Tannoy, as I was called up to get a prize – I had won the women's over-fifty age group. But as I went up to the commentators, Steve Trew and Ian Pettitt, to collect my medal, they looked at my times: 1 hour, 15 minutes for the 1500-metre swim. 'My God, we must be able to improve on that,' said Steve, and 'If I can get Rocco Forte's time down, I can improve yours.' That was the beginning of Steve's long-lasting support and friendship.

One day, early in 2003, I had a casual but life-changing conversation. Talking to my Serpentine friend Maria, I was bemoaning my appalling swimming. She suggested that I tried a duathlon. I had no idea what a duathlon was, but I looked it up on the British Triathlon website. Maria was going down to Swindon to do a duathlon in May, so I signed up too. I was totally relaxed – a new fun experience – no pressures at all.

We registered and as the start time approached I noticed that everyone's right legs were marked with a letter of the alphabet – it carried no significance for me, just a black letter on my calf. I was feeling pretty apprehensive as we lined up on a country track with about thirty other women at the appointed time. I hovered towards the back of what I now knew to be the over-50s group. Then I heard a very confident woman who seemed to know everyone say loudly, 'Do you realise there is an L with us?' I looked down, and sure enough there was a big L on my fat calf. I lacked the confidence to identify myself, so I kept my head down. Scanning other calf muscles in front of me it slowly dawned that 'L' indicated my age group, 60–65 years. I was the oldest woman there.

So on 18 May 2003, aged sixty, I completed my first duathlon through the lovely soft woods and countryside of Wiltshire. I was confronted by the unique challenges of a duathlon – a 10k run, then the 40k bike and finally another

5k run – for the first time, and I loved it. There is nothing to compare with the difficulty of starting that second run, on tired legs, aching muscles struggling to change gear, legs that feel like jelly needing persuasion to do anything other than a gentle plodding jog. I had done four marathons by now, but this was a totally new and challenging experience.

Somehow, I finished, albeit towards the back of the pack. However, as I went to get my finisher's medal I realised I was indeed the only L, the only one in the 60–65 age range. Another competitor asked me if I had registered to compete for the GB team in that age group. This race had apparently been a qualifying event for those seeking to represent Great Britain in the European or World Championships. At the time I had no idea what he meant, or the rule that if I was proposing to use this race as a qualifying event, then I should have indicated my intentions when I entered the race. But the officials of British Triathlon accepted the confusion of an elderly 'L', and allowed me to sign up – as a member of the GB team for the Duathlon World Championships in Affoltern, Switzerland, in late August.

A day or so later the reality of what I had committed to hit me. The thought of competing in a world championship was all the more daunting because I knew I had qualified only because I was the sole 60–65 athlete to enter the Swindon duathlon. After some reflection, I decided I had to do the GB team justice, and achieve the best I could. For that, I needed the assistance and discipline of a training programme. I again approached Brian Welsh of Just Sweat No Tears, who had joined us as a triathlon coach on the Serpentine Lanzarote trip.

Brian gave me a plan and I reported to him weekly. This was a new discipline for me, but one in which I was reasonably compliant. Brian lived up in Derbyshire too, so that fitted well with my trips back to the Peak District. Very quickly I got to know other members of his local networks, and occasionally I went out with them in the beautiful, hilly countryside. I found a great run course near Blackclough, where I could do my timed hill sprints. One day I made a stunning discovery. Lap after lap I pushed myself to the very limit uphill and was able to make only a difference of seconds over a half-kilometre, but over the next few laps I realised that, running downhill, I could save almost a minute if I really pushed it. I could make up more time running faster downhill than I lost going uphill, and I was saving energy at the same time. I developed far more confidence in downhill, though, with hindsight, that may not have helped the arthritis in my knees. I also developed a lovely hilly time trial on the bike, riding a circle around Blackclough. In those days I managed it in under an hour – it now takes significantly longer.

August 2003 arrived, and my first GB trip. Ordering and buying the kit is expensive, and then there is the further step of getting your name printed on the back of the tri-suit. With its ten letters, Brocklesby was more expensive than my maiden name Higgins. So out to Switzerland and the long coach trip up to Affoltern, the smallest city in Switzerland and five hundred metres above sea level. Once settled into the hotel, the first sortie was to the Parade of Nations – and new friends. The pasta party followed, with most abstemiously rejecting alcohol until John, another GB team member, suggested a beer – a very welcome idea. The atmosphere over supper that night was tense but friendly.

Steve came out the following day on his bike to support me, or, more accurately, to get in some serious cycling mileage before his first Ironman – but it was great to have him there. The morning of the race, 31 August 2003, was unforgettable. We were up really early to find it had poured with

rain throughout the night. I managed a sort of breakfast and
it was still pitch dark. We were transported down to the large
marquee close to the start of the race. It was only just dawn
when all the women went off at seven-thirty. The men were
luckier, starting two hours later, in the light and without the
rain. What a memorable day. The run course was hilly, starting with an incline out of transition and then a steady slope
up and further up. The course didn't dry out until midway,
by which time we were on the second run.

I had been looking forward to the four-lap bike leg but I
soon wilted on the first steady climb and then the downhill
bends. I clung cautiously to the edge of the road, braking at
every turn on the wet roads, looking down over the steep
drop to the fields below. Closed roads were still a relatively
new phenomenon to me and everyone was overtaking
me. Then suddenly the shout of another Serpie, Rebecca,
swooping down and lapping me: 'Come on, Eddie, it is
absolutely great, no cars – enjoy!' and she was gone, far more
aerodynamically positioned than I was, down and away into
the distance below. Wow. I eased off my brakes and found
Rebecca was dead right. It was great. I could control the
bike even when going fast downhill. I began to really revel
in it, and found for the first time that climbing back up was
just something you had to endure for the joy of another race
downhill. I was aware that people were dropping out with
varying degrees of hypothermia – we apparently raced in sub
fifty-degree weather. I had no idea of their ages, but I knew
that I was overtaking women on the side, very cold women
in their USA gear. I learned later they came from Florida
and were clearly unused to such conditions, and unprepared
for such a brutal Swiss mountain course. By the final lap the
sun was peeking through the clouds and the conditions were
noticeably better. Still one hour and fifty minutes on the bike

was not a bad time on a tough course in tough conditions, and apparently, we were told later, it was actually two kilometres longer than the standard 40k.

When I finally got back into transition I knew I was in second place as I dropped the bike, changed back into my running shoes and pushed myself up the slope and out of transition. There was no way I could start running until at least four hundred metres in, and then I faced a slow, slow drag up the hill again – but just two laps this time. I overtook a few people on the upwards slope, but didn't know their age group. But there at the bottom of the penultimate lap was Steve saying 'Mum, I think you are in the lead; I think you are going to get gold!' I did get gold, in 3 hours, 11 minutes. Of the original eight competitors in my age group, only three of us had finished.

That evening there was a party and awards celebrations. I had never experienced anything like it before – coaches, team managers and professionals all in one place. It was a great atmosphere and I appreciated for the first time the camaraderie and that it mattered to the GB team how many gold, silver and bronze medals had been won. As I was called up to the podium and stood on the top deck, it added to the GB medals tally. It was absolutely unbelievable that I was an 'oldie' age-group world champion who four months earlier hadn't even known of the existence of duathlons.

What celebrations, what a fantastic experience and what great new friends – GB and worldwide. The age group fraternity is great and Affoltern was to be the first of many World Duathlon Championships for me.

Two years later I entered the World Long-Distance Duathlon in Barcis, Italy. I had briefly met the world champion Benny Vansteelant before the race, and at the point that I had finished my first run, and was making my tortuously

slow way up an endless climb, Benny, bombing downhill
towards the finish, looked up and shouted out encouragement
to me. He was equally enthusiastic as he congratulated me
at the awards ceremony. He had won the race overall and I
was second in my age group. What a heartbreakingly sad loss
when he was killed a few years later.

That race was significant as I met my future mentor and
friend Annie Emmerson. Annie had won multiple races
round the world, and was the world number one duathlete.
There with Michelle Parsons, those two professionals occu-
pied a totally different world to me. Slim, brilliant athletes
with very posh sunglasses – we were a world apart.

I knew Annie and Michelle were also going to the World
Championships in Newcastle, Australia, later that year. With
that in mind, we discussed the possibility of Annie helping
me. It was a fortuitous connection. I have never looked back
and Annie's indomitably encouraging, positive spirit has been
there for me now for eleven years.

It was a fantastic experience to spend time with Annie
in what was to be her last race as a professional athlete. Her
mum had travelled to Australia too for that final duathlon,
which she completed in a staggering 2 hours, 12 minutes. It
took me 3 hours and 1 minute – although I did win gold in
my 60–64 age group!

As well as coaching, Annie now commentates on triathlon
for the BBC. She's seen many of the barriers that those who
are new to the sport are facing. Asked what the challenges
she faced in taking on the training of an older woman, Annie
replied:

'To be honest, there were fewer than with some people –
Eddie is pretty straightforward and she doesn't overthink
things like some younger athletes do. She is always up for
a challenge. Nothing is too hard for her. When you coach

someone older, you worry more about their health and the impact on the joints. But Eddie's a bit of a phenomenon and she's worn pretty well. The challenges I faced were keeping her in one piece, and trying to make sure she didn't over train, ensuring she achieves her goals. I really can't say there were any bad challenges, only the over training.'

Varella in Italy was the venue of another duathlon – a long-distance European championship. I learned a hard lesson there – I arrived late, only the day before the event, with no time to adjust, check out any of the route, or just chill out. Boring and tense though such a few days can be, it is a more crucial part of competitions than I had appreciated. I won't forget being told off by a more experienced teammate, who was fearful that I wouldn't be able to do my best and earn a medal for the GB team. As the 'oldie' female in the team, I steadily became aware that I could be a valuable commodity. If there weren't many in my age group I had a higher chance of medalling than the forty-somethings in their huge and massively competitive age groups.

And so, sport wise, it was on to Rimini and the World Duathlon Championships of 2008. I was now sixty-six, and a few younger contenders were coming on to the over-sixty-five scene. There was an acceptance, undoubtedly evidenced by research, that, as you age through the five-year span, the younger ones have the advantage. They had had some unseasonably bad weather in Italy, and when the age-group men had gone off on the Saturday, the afternoon before my race, many of them had punctured and given up. But by the time we women went on the Sunday morning, the sun was shining, the roads had been swept and cleaned and it was a wonderfully friendly international group. I was a relatively new girl on the block but knew the opposition, and deferred massively to the German competitor in my age group, who I knew from previous events was a far stronger runner than me. The first run 10k was straightforward, the bike was six laps and then the 5k run. I came in second in my age group and congratulated my German opponent who had come first, pleased for her and pleased for myself.

And then, that evening when results were put up on the hotel noticeboard, I saw I was placed first – my poor German friend had stopped her bike ride a lap short and gone out onto the run. I didn't see her after the race, and when we met again the following year there was an anxious moment of hesitation – do I make a joke about her ability to count to six? I did, and she responded with great humour and affection. It was so easy to get it wrong on multi-lap events, in the days before high-tech GPS wearables and accurate distance measurement.

My duathlon career to date had seen me win three gold medals in World Championships in Switzerland, Australia and Italy. All were great adventures, which allowed me to explore the world in a focused way, meet fabulous people and have fun. How very, very, very lucky I am.

6

Things rarely go the way you think they will

Race across America (RAAM) is described as one the most respected and longest running endurance sports events in the world, the pinnacle of athletic achievement not only in cycling circles but in the greater sporting community as well. In 1982, four individuals raced from the Santa Monica Pier in Los Angeles to the Empire State Building in New York City. Relay-team riding was added in 1992. Those teams, in theory, made the event accessible to any reasonably fit cyclist.

The organisers say – through rose-colour spectacles, in my view – that 'The Race inspires everyone who has been a part of it – racer, crew, staff and fans alike. RAAM is the true test of speed, endurance, strength and camaraderie, the ideal combination of work and fun!' They add, 'There is no race that matches the distance, terrain and weather, no other event that tests a team's spirit from beginning to end.' That is certainly not an understatement.

The route has altered slightly over the years, but it now

crosses twelve states, with 30,770 metres of climbing. Only 15 per cent of the racers are women. The RAAM rules are very tight. The route is strictly detailed, the distances prescribed and the regular staging points at which the competitors have to phone in and report their position are well defined. The riders need to have light behind them from a support car during the hours of dusk and dark. There are relay teams of eight, teams of four and two, and – the real heroes – the solo riders. The solo riders start off earlier, with twelve days to complete the 3014 miles. Four-person teams have nine days. Cut-off times are soul-destroyingly rigid as my first coach, Brian Welsh, will testify from his first solo ride in 2014. Heartbreakingly, he arrived at the finish just two hours over the limit. Having had barely any sleep for twelve days, he ended up with a DNF (Did Not Finish) against his name. However, he has recently completed the solo, unsupported Trans Am Bike Race, and in 2018 he plans to do RAAM again in a four-person relay team, with the aim of setting a new age-group record.

Back in 2006 I had been asked by Brian if I would be pre-pared to crew for his mixed team: three men and a woman. He assured me I'd be an asset to the crew, as 'You can manage without much sleep'. I certainly hadn't appreciated what I was letting myself in for, or that coping with sleep depriva-tion is key. Each team in RAAM has a support crew, riding in two to three vehicles, depending on the size of the team. The crew size varies too, and may be driving, map-reading, providing food and water, or able to undertake mechanical repairs or medical aid. During the night, a vehicle is required to follow each rider to ensure their safety, and to give the rider security and light ahead of them.

I had joined up with Brian's Just Sweat No Tears team at Oceanside in California with my own new bike, confident that I would have plenty of opportunities to get out on the road myself. I had come on to join the RAAM team from a brilliant two-week holiday in Australia, where Kate, her husband John and son Ben were living for a year in Brisbane. As part of a reciprocal scheme, just prior to consultancy posts, Kate was working as a paediatrician, but was able at weekends to enjoy the beauty of the Sunshine Coast, and the Great Barrier Reef. For the first time I had bought cleats to fit onto my cycling shoes, that fitted into the new pedals. I recall trying them out on the first day, alongside a river in Brisbane. It was fine fitting the shoes into the pedals as I started off, but 'de-cleating' and getting off the bike was another matter. Embarrassingly, I fell off – the first of many, many such experiences. But despite a sore shoulder, John and I did the Noosa Triathlon on the Sunshine Coast and loved it.

It turned out that the thought of getting in any further bike riding in RAAM was optimistic. Apart from a short one-hour ride, my bike remained tied to the Winnebago. However, it was a valuable asset as it was plundered for essential spare parts by the racers.

As a crew member for Brian's team, I learned that RAAM is all about the crew and logistics. Even prima donna riders have to accept rapidly that they depend totally on a well-functioning crew. Ideally, a four-person team has a Winnebago and two support vehicles. The team is divided into two pairs, each with their own support vehicle, and the generally accepted model is that two people alternately ride an hour each for eight hours. Whilst Rider 1 is riding, Rider 2 is in the support vehicle following closely behind. After an hour the support vehicle overtakes and drives a mile or so up ahead to get Rider 2's bike off the rack and Rider 2 ready at the roadside. Rider 2 is then touched by Rider 1 as they arrive, and Rider 2 can then speed off. The support vehicle loads up Rider 1 and their bike before going back up the road to Rider 2. The aim is for optimum efficiency, a brilliantly smooth handover in the quickest time possible.

The route is planned to enable about 8 hours riding with a fixed, identified meeting point at the end. At the end of a stint, the two teams swap over. Rider 3 sets off and Rider 4 gets into the second support vehicle. Riders 1 and 2 get into the Winnebago to eat and rest. The driver and navigator of the support vehicles often swap over at the same time. Sleep is often unlikely as the Winnebago departs, overtakes the riders and drives on to the next designated handover stop, some eight bike-riding hours ahead. Although it is a team relay, the two riders see remarkably little of the other pair and indeed they see little of the other riders in the race, aside from occasionally being overtaken by an eight-person team, or passing a duo or solo competitor.

After the first day or two, positions in RAAM tend to be relatively fixed, with not much overtaking of other teams or individuals. It can be a lonely journey. Frustratingly, our sole means of communicating with our other crew members were large intercom devices that rarely worked. In 2006, mobile signals were non-existent in the Midwest.

But as far as the crew is concerned, their life is far, far harder. Sleep deprivation begins to kick in after a couple of days and without the release of getting any physical exercise, tensions rise, group dynamics change and nutrition gets ever worse. The physical and emotional demands on the crew are massive. Logistics are such that the crew also tends to operate in pairs and there is nothing worse, as other teams had found in the past, than navigating or driving for sixteen hours with a partner who is erratic, or shattered. Perhaps worse still is the knowledge that at night, when, exhausted and sleep-deprived, you are driving only a couple of metres behind your rider. If you should fall asleep and lose control you could kill them. Years on, I can still picture myself at the wheel, dangerously tired, driving at night behind one of our riders, Kevin, who was swooping down a steep woodland hill at an alarming pace. He was totally dependent on the light from the RV I was driving. Matching his increasing speed, and avoiding crashing into him was a scary challenge.

In central regions of the States the road is straight as a die for mile after mile after mile and it is so easy to lose concentration. As you pass through the occasional town, you could understand why apparently less than 20 per cent of America citizens had a passport. Graphically you could see the extent to which out-of-town malls ruled, with a total absence of public transport. No wonder car ownership was essential, and oil and gas so vital to the economy.

Frustratingly, you drive through places you've heard of and dreamt of visiting. We passed signs to Las Vegas, or famous mining towns, with no opportunity to stop and sightsee. In 2006 the RAAM route went down next to the Mexican border and into a crater of similar depth to the Grand Canyon. I don't think I have ever been as scared as navigating on the inside edge of the Winnebago on the right side of the road, twisting steeply downhill, looking over the drop so far below.

Our Winnebago had space to sleep four, but safety instructions insisted that no one should lie down in the bed over the cab when the vehicle is in motion, removing one potential sleeping option for tired cyclists or crew whilst we were on the move. Only in a static vehicle could riders or crew get some quality sleep. Shattered one day, I climbed into my sleeping bag and lay down on the bed at the back of the van, next to another body. When the driver braked violently, I flew off the high bed onto the floor and slid the full length of the vehicle.

It was an eventful race. Nearing the end, some two hundred miles short of the finish line in Atlantic City, I was driving and making a left turn at traffic lights, just two or three feet behind Russell, our well-built, six-foot-tall rider. Suddenly he was hit by a vehicle turning across him – he sailed up into the air, across our bonnet and landed on the ground on my side of the car. With screeching brakes, all the traffic at the junction came to a standstill. But with great presence of mind (or ultimate competitiveness) Brian, the cyclist in the back of the support vehicle I was driving, jumped out, grabbed his bike and rode on. It was a long, long time before we caught him up.

We rapidly gathered Russell up at the crossroads, amazingly with only a broken finger, a very sore leg, and a smashed-up bike. I drove off with Russell in the car, to catch up with Brian as quickly as possible. A few miles later, with sirens screaming behind us, we were forced to stop. The police had interviewed the angry car driver that had collided with Russell. His car was damaged, so both he and the police had set off in hot pursuit of us. Full statements were taken. I think the fact that I was an older, female English driver protected us from the litigation that could have followed, having 'driven off from the scene of an accident'.

The route into the finish at Atlantic City was a horrendous three-lane motorway, with a very narrow bike lane. It was very scary for both cyclist and accompanying vehicle. The finish line was a mile or so further out from the ceremonial finish, so all four riders – even Russell with his painful injured leg – could ride to the finish, and get the reception they so justly deserved. They finished seven hours before the cut-off time.

We were so eagerly waiting that first drink, and a sit-down meal. We had been dreaming of little else for several days. Alcohol is banned for riders and crew throughout RAAM.

We found our four-bed hotel room. Any bed at all was a total luxury, and I lay down whilst others had a shower first. The next thing I knew it was eleven hours later. They had all pushed me, shouted at me, shoved me, trying to wake me, and finally given up and gone out to celebrate without me. Such was my state of exhaustion.

After crewing for the Just Sweat No Tears team in 2006, I wanted to have a go myself, in a four-person team. Brian planned to do it with his wife Stacey – just the two of them in a relay, raising funds for our charity, Parents for Children.

Our team for the 2008 RAAM slowly formed, from four female members of Serpentine Running Club, and out of the blue a fifth person, Hilary (Hils) Webber, contacted us through Brian, as she had heard about the formation of this older women's team. We put out a request for a team name over our Serpentine club e-group. A variety of suggestions flowed back, some less than polite! We settled on the Serpentine Golden Girls, who, if ages were taken at the end of the year we raced would have averaged just over sixty. But, sadly, taken on our ages at the time of the race, we were oh so marginally under sixty, and in competition with another women's four-person team with an average age of fifty to sixty. It wasn't about prizes, but more about reputation and achievement as a team.

We set about assembling our crew and our vehicles. We knew we needed a bike expert, a physio, and six more crew members who could cope with sleep deprivation to be drivers. We advertised on a physio/health college noticeboard for a physio or masseuse to join the crew. I knew from my crewing experience that stiffness crept in big time by day three. When Naomi, who was also a paramedic, contacted us, we couldn't believe our luck. She did her massages for the four of us in some unbelievable settings. Richard was our bike expert, and we were so fortunate that his partner Gemma was able to persuade Hyundai to donate the use of two support vehicles for our RAAM team.

Everyone else was related to or knew our riders, or another member of the crew. We were so very grateful to them for giving up two weeks' holiday and supporting us so brilliantly. One crew member recalls chatting to me at a New Year's Eve party, and waking up on New Year's Day to find he was on the Serpentine Golden Girls RAAM crew. Recruiting the crew and preparing them for what is to come is so important. Even with all my years of experience of group dynamics and individual personalities and histories, you can still underesti-mate how people behave under sleep-deprived pressure.

We signed up as a four-woman team: Margaret Sills, Hilary Walker, Hilary (Hils) Webber and me, with Ros Young as our understudy. At sixty-five, I was the oldest. Starting at Oceanside and finishing in Annapolis in Maryland, the 2008 RAAM route crossed the Rockies and the desert plains.

The strong advice from experienced RAAM riders is to train up five people, as you never know what will happen in the six months leading up to the June start. We will always be grateful to Ros for going all the way through our training, prepared to be a rider in the event of a problem for any one of the four riders, and in the end acting as crew chief. Once the race has started no substitutes are allowed – an understandable but frustrating rule.

As it happened, the demands on Ros were even greater, because in late 2007 I was still recovering from having my appendix removed in the August. I was reasonably com-pliant with the medical advice by not doing much training post-surgery, so it was December by the time I got back on the bike and began to do any serious mileage. There must have been times when the other three surveyed the potential competence of their oldest team member and wondered if she would make it to the start line, or, worse still, would she be a liability for them in not playing her full part, either at the right speed or in terms of hours on the bike?

RAAM is costly. Paying for vehicle hire, rider and crew fares from the UK, overnight hotel stays at the beginning and the end, and fuel and food throughout, we estimated that with the kind support of Hyundai for the hire of the vehicles, it would be roughly twenty-thousand pounds: five thousand pounds for each of us. Our crew was brilliant, even though they must have regretted their decision to join us on many, many occasions.

Although more expensive, it is more efficient for the riders and night-time changes if the team has two support vehicles rather than one, plus the Winnebago. But with a crew of eight, and a team of four, peaceful, deep sleep for everyone is erratic, and often far too brief. The crew are effectively driving or navigating for sixteen hours out of twenty-four, the riders doing three eight-hour stints in every forty-eight hours. Sleep deprivation is inevitable, and all the bike train-ing, and team building doesn't really prepare you for that eight-day span. Dynamics between the riders matter far less than between the crew as you rarely see the other two for more than a fleeting 'hi' and you are off, one riding, the other close behind in the support vehicle. The riders also have the benefit of riding, getting rid of any tensions, enjoying the fantastic scenery or the smells and sounds of the darkness, the animals that cross in front, lights in the far, far distance of straight roads for mile after mile. For the crew, as I knew all too well, there is no such respite.

Getting some balance in nutrition and sleep is vital for crew and riders. The other sponsorship that Just Sweat No Tears had when I crewed for them was from High5. I had always used their caffeine-loaded EXTRA nutrition, in the form of energy drinks and gels. I recall the looks of horror of one of the others when I announced that, on the personal advice of the High5 directors, Tim and Mick Atkinson, I would be taking two gels ten minutes before each of my one-hour stints, until I got to my last hour, when I took non-caffeinated gels so that, after some solid food, I would be better able to sleep. It was certainly a high caffeine level, but I had trained with it over several years. Then, in the carefully designed plan, after riding for an hour I would have a peanut butter sandwich and a coffee back in the support vehicle. When we finished the eight hours the crew would then have pasta or baked potatoes waiting for us in the Winnebago.

We overtook several solo and duo teams, including Brian and Stacey. Both strong riders, we ended up close to them for some while, with the opportunities to cheer them on, and chat to their crew, recognising that as individuals they were cycling twice as far as any of our team of four, with far less time to sleep.

I was so, so impressed by the phenomenal athlete and multi-Ironman competitor Jim Rees, from Hertfordshire, who was a solo rider in 2008. We had met him before we set out and seen a film about his ride the previous year, when he'd only just made the cut-off time by eight minutes. His neck had been acutely painful for most of the race, strapped up with some form of tubing to keep it in a straight line. Clearly in distress, his efforts over the twelve days were inspirational. So when I caught up with him in 2008, it was a privilege to ride alongside him for a while, learning more of the origins of his Team Inspiration and his motivational work with children. 'We are all built for greatness – what mark are you going to make?' was his perspective. It was indeed inspirational that he again managed to finish before the solo cut-off time.

RAAM permits bike-riding with an earphone in one ear. My son had shown me how to put two of my CDs onto my iPod, and then left me to download the rest. Somehow I didn't find the time to do it, so ended up with just the two albums' worth of Billy Joel to listen to. He is a long-time favourite, but for forty-eight hours of riding, it was just him and me, 'Uptown Girl', 'Only the Good Die Young', 'It's Still Rock and Roll to Me', 'Allentown Way', my favourite, 'Keeping the Faith', and the slower beat of 'Piano Man' (when I realised that my own cycling cadence slowed down too). I was going to either love or hate Billy Joel for the rest of my life. Fortunately, it was the former, and I have now been to see him live in concerts in Dublin, Wembley and New York, all evoking powerful and fabulous memories of different scenes of RAAM.

I was partnered by Hils, who is a far better hill-climber than me; she stoically did more of the climbing. Our satnav showed us when hills were imminent and she certainly went out early sometimes and did more than her fair share of climbing. It was just not fair that she had done more climbing but I had the luck of coming down, and down, from the Rockies for one whole brilliant and scenic hour.

Travelling west to east means riders see only sunrises, no sunsets. But those sunrises were spectacular, with the glimpse of light on the wide horizon of the plains and then, slowly, over my hour of riding the dawn would rise. We riders really were the lucky ones. I think I was the only rider to see a sunset. On one brief left-hand turn I could see, over to my left, the most spectacular colours over the plains. Then, a mile or so further on, the route took a right-hand turn and the sunset was again behind me.

We were lucky with the wind too. The prevailing wind was behind us for the first few hundred miles, but then it turned and suddenly the wind was in my face. It was really hard going. My speed dropped dramatically for a mile or so, and then, suddenly, the route took a right turn, and the wind was behind us again. What an incredible relief.

My best and abiding memory of RAAM was one very special dawn. I took over in Utah when it was only just getting light. The rocks of the National Park on either side were a shimmering pink colour, the natural rock formation loomed larger and larger on the right side and a huge Indian reservation monument, the Navajo Nation Tribal Park was on the left. I cycled silently through the pink sandy desert scenery. As it got lighter the support vehicle was able to drop back a bit so I was totally on my own – alone on my bike with my thoughts and, as ever, Billy Joel helping me to 'Keep the Faith', yet feeling totally safe and supported by the team. Life doesn't get any better. I was indeed the lucky one, the only sadness being that Phil wasn't with me to share such a dramatic and beautiful experience.

Asking the others for their memorable moments, Hils remembered me cycling in the Colorado Mountains. As a mascot, and keeping me company throughout, I was carrying on my back one of the hundreds of Buildabear teddies that had been donated to Parents for Children. Hils watched from the support vehicle behind as an eagle swooped down on my bear, and she imagined me being lifted and carried off by the eagle, still pedalling!

None of us had anticipated the contrasting temperatures on our journey, from the desert to the mountains. One day, Hilary and Margaret had finished their stint and had handed over to Hils and me. Hils had gone off first to ride, so the three of us had a few minutes to speak before I and the support vehicle went after her. Margaret and Hilary had brought a snowball down from the mountain summit to show us how cold it had been – we had been fast asleep during the latter part of their eight-hour stint, and had had no idea. By now, we were down at sea level. Hils and I never did experience the extreme cold temperatures of RAAM.

It may have been on that occasion or a subsequent one – days merged – that, twenty minutes into Hils's stint, I got a phone call from Hilary: 'Eddie – do you need a bike to ride RAAM?' My bike had come down from the Winnebago but I had forgotten to load it into the support vehicle and so it remained at the roadside. Hilary will always remind me of this incident if ever I mention how she incurred us a penalty point for failing to put a foot down on the ground at the white line of a crossroads somewhere in the isolated outback of the USA. Fancy not seeing the RAAM marshal skulking in the hedgerow in the middle of nowhere! RAAM punishes such offences by issuing penalty points, so time has to be served in the next penalty box along the route. Suffice to say that only one of us has a T-shirt denoting accrued penalty points, and there are photos of Hilary sitting for fifteen minutes in the penalty box, the rest of us watching and laughing.

On day six we hit typhoon territory. Hils and I were riding. The skies ever blackening, the silence was eerie. No rain yet. With our driver and navigator, we were listening to the local radio in the support vehicle as Hils rode ahead of us. We could see the dramatic black typhoon shape in the far distance, and heard the forecast, accurately predicting the movement of the typhoon directly towards us. The dangers of typhoons were being vividly described on the radio, memories being relayed of huge iron statues being lifted by the storm and dumped in fields a mile away. Not a little scared by the local knowledge we were listening to, the four of us decided to pull into a large rural Walmart and allow the

Winnebago and the other support vehicle to catch us up. We then shared the decision to cut our leg short and rest up for a couple of hours until the storm passed.

We relaxed in Walmart until the rest of the group caught up with us and we did a handover. Unfortunately, the delay enabled the rain to catch up with us too. Poor Margaret rode off in appalling conditions, with Hilary in the support vehicle. Meanwhile another couple of teams had just ridden on, ignoring the risks of the typhoon, almost certainly without the 'benefit' of hearing the local radio racking up the crisis. They had stayed ahead of the rainstorm. It was a difficult call, and one, with the benefit of hindsight, we got wrong.

I'm not sure that any of us were really prepared for the mountains and the climbing that we hit in the last two days of the race. By now we were far, far more tired and muscles were screaming. With amazing endurance, Hils again did far more than her share of those climbs. This may have contributed to one of our very few tension-driven incidents, when I stood roadside at the top of the hill with my bike, waiting to start, but Hils went riding on past me and the support vehicle. Immediately, we all understood that having done that endless climb for an hour in the hot sun, Hils needed to have some recovery time on the flat or downhill road. It was amazing that similar incidents didn't happen more often, with four mature but nevertheless driven individualist profiles. We wouldn't have been facing the challenges of RAAM without those characteristics.

And so to the final miles. Margaret took on the last leg to the finish line, glamorously placed in a shopping mall car park on the outskirts of Annapolis. There we had a chance to re-group and the four of us rode in, just after midnight, to finish in 8 days, 5 hours and 19 minutes. Despite the hour of the night, there was a reception team, interviews and photos, and my son Steve and his wife Jane, who had come all that way to celebrate with us.

Brian and Stacey finished shortly after, in 8 days and 17 hours. They were only the second mixed pair to make the nine-day time cut-off in thirty years of the race.

We remain eternally grateful to all our crew. It is not easy to be fully prepared for the experience of RAAM, the sleep deprivation, group dynamics, lack of opportunity to be physically active, not to mention demanding and at times unreasonable riders. Reflecting, what did each of us get out of the race, and would we ever do it again? Perhaps suffice to say that we are thinking seriously about 2019 as an eleventh-anniversary ride – with an average age of over seventy!

7

Dreams don't always live up
to your expectations

B ack in May, before RAAM, I had gone out to Lanzarote
to support Steve, who was racing the Ironman there. His
wife Jane and I became adept at driving or cycling around
the island, so that on race day we could get out to see Steve
on the bike on four occasions, stop for coffee and cakes at
El Pastelito, the amazing German bakery in Tahiche, and
make it back to Puerto del Carmen for the run. This is when
support really counts – when exhaustion creeps in, energy
depletes and a smiling and encouraging personalised support
can reinvigorate, or just enable someone to keep going, keep
pounding and keep smiling. It was that day in 2008 when I
finally decided I would have a go myself.

I loved the island, I loved the route and I knew from being
there many times to cheer Steve that the support on the run
along the main coastal bar and shopping road in Puerto del
Carman was fantastic. And at the end, there was the legendary
Kenneth Gasque to welcome home every single competitor,

from those who finished in under nine hours right through to those trying to beat the midnight cut-off. Kenneth had been the first Dane to compete in the Ironman World Championship in Kona, Hawaii, and went on, in 1992, to set up and manage Ironman Lanzarote. Assisted by my good friend Isabelle, he has been the race director ever since.

Even for an anxious open-water swimmer like me, the sea swim at Ironman Lanzarote is great. You do two laps of a rectangle parallel to the coastline. The water is crystal clear, with loads of fabulously coloured fish below. A long, long row of small buoys on the far side of the rectangle means that at any point you can stop, hold on, have a breather, get better sighting and set off again. Open-water swimming is all about swimming in as straight a line as possible, thus minimising the distance swum. I had learned to lift my head just enough every six strokes to sight on a boat, or a tree or building in the distance, but that long row of buoys was far more helpful. If I was ever going to do an Ironman, this, I told myself, was the place. And the real bonus was that Steve was prepared to do it again. I knew he would be far ahead of me, but just the knowledge that he was out there on the course or in a nearby bar at the end would be enough.

And so it was to be. Goals were set and training done – on the bike and the swimming over far greater distances than I had ever done in my life. Swimming 1.5k had been my absolute limit. Could I really swim 3.8 kilometres in the Atlantic Ocean? I turned to Annie Emmerson for encouragement, support and, above all, her belief that I could do an Ironman-distance triathlon, even at my age. She gave me a weekly training programme that I would try to follow – although over our occasional evening glass of wine together she would challenge my adherence to her plans.

The swim was, and remains, the greatest challenge for

me. I had had lessons from Dan Bullock from Swim for Tri, and joined several of their weekly training sessions, and even swim camps. I asked Dan to reflect on my swim training and any lessons he had learned from teaching an older person with no swimming background:

> As far as natural talent goes, this wasn't really the case for Eddie. Shoulders made of concrete were going to be a real hindrance to getting any kind of upper-body rotation and arm recovery. As part of her regular weekly training, yoga and stretching were encouraged – these would help mobilise her strong upper body. The strength she had developed to keep her trunk rigid while running, her first sport, was impressive, but in order for her to mobilise and streamline, we needed to add the ability to relax and increase her range of motion. Upper-body rotation through the long axis of the body while keeping the head still took months. Eventually, with a lot of practice and the sort of determination that distinguishes Elite Competitors, these skills came and progress was made. What was lacking in natural talent was offset with tenacity. I have met few with such an appetite and desire to improve.
>
> The general drills programme Eddie followed in her own time were restricting incorrect movements, encouraging correct movements and, perhaps most importantly, interrupting the 'auto-pilot' movements that had been creating inefficiencies and slowing her down. She was moving from the stage of 'unconscious incompetence' towards 'conscious competence', which required a lot of thought, effort and diligence in creating correct pathways that reduced drag and created propulsion.
>
> Frustration levels ran pretty high when we first started work on front crawl. The water was too cold, the goggles

leaked or the chlorine was too high. 'Why does it need to be so complicated?' was often asked. Interestingly, the fact that Eddie was quickly becoming a better cyclist was not helping matters. 'If I can be fast at this new sport of biking then why not this swimming nonsense?' Comparisons to learning a new language or a musical instrument as an older adult fell on deaf ears. I hoped Eddie would have the patience to see through another winter and keep at it. We were working hard to keep her motivated, challenged and inspired. It was not easy to convince her that taking a step back from her fitness sessions to work on technique would help in the longer term. Of course, she was not about to become unfit while biking and running so much, but it is highly counter-intuitive for someone with a Championship mindset to be told to step back a little, take it easy and be patient. Keeping track of progress and setting new challenges was key.

At this point, it was not possible for Eddie to contemplate swimming as active recovery – to be able to go and have a nice relaxed easy swim to recover from a bike or run session. When this did become possible it was a real breakthrough in terms of enjoying relaxed swimming – the act of swimming, even very slowly, had been exhausting. Eddie struggled with physical limitations and restrictions, as well as a lack of confidence and coordination in the water. The combination of physical and mental obstacles proved to be one of the toughest challenges to overcome.

While friends, club coaches and teammates all meant well with advice and suggestions, the information overload was hindering progress. Most swimmers learning good technique in their adult years find the process can be quite overwhelming and need to get their main technical coaching from one consistent source. That is not to say there is only one way to go about improving your training and that we have cracked it. Far from it. But if many voices are adding comments at different stages of progression, this causes issues.

Club swimming sessions may be a great, social part of weekly training and may be a great way to increase some levels of swim-specific fitness, but there are not that many chances to work precisely on technique. Broadly speaking, most swimmers are focused on keeping up with everyone else in their lane and often sacrifice almost any amount of technique in order to do that. For Eddie, the desire to make personal progress was stronger than the desire to keep up with other swimmers, so one-to-one sessions became a bigger part of the routine.

The increase in weekly distances swum meant that certain body parts needed strengthening to cope with this increase. A dryland routine was introduced ahead of each session to mobilise key swimming muscle groups and start the warm-up sequence allowing her to enter the water 'warm'. Working with Annie Emmerson has been of great help in coordinating a full plan of attack for getting Eddie race ready.

Despite all the confidence-building help and advice from Annie and Dan, and the familiarity of Lanzarote, it felt very different to be going out to be a participant in my first Ironman, compared with playing the support role. Steve and I arrived at Club La Santa for registration and it all seemed very low-key, with several friendly and familiar faces from our annual Serpentine trips, many clearly surprised I was an entrant. Then, as I collected my race pack, I could see great red marker pen across my name, and was asked, 'Please could you go just over there to talk to the press team.' I realised I must have been the oldest female competitor they had ever had, and I was to be one of three or four competitors they were planning to follow for their film. I was interviewed the day before the race, and filmed racking my bike that evening, then anxiously arriving in the morning as dawn was breaking.

Getting all the bags sorted for an Ironman is a logistical nightmare: one for the swim, one for the bike, one for the run and then a 'street bag' for the belongings you'll need at the end. After sticking race numbers on to the bags, my helmet and my bike, it was time to take everything down to the transition area. In race week, part of the high street is converted to an endless fenced-off transition area. As you go through the entrance, helmet on, numbers checked, bike brakes checked, the panic rises. Am I mad? Then another dilemma: how far should I let the tyres down, just in case the late-evening heat causes expansion and a blow-out?

Finally, it was back to the hotel for a silent supper. Advice states no heavy carb-loading as it could impede the few hours of sleep ahead. I do usually sleep well, despite the panic. The alarm was set for 4 a.m., allowing me time to finish breakfast an hour and a half ahead of the race start. Further details would be too much information – just bear in mind that by 6.45 a.m. I would be zipped up and locked into a wetsuit.

At 6 a.m., street bag in hand, wetsuit, hat and goggles at the ready, it was back down to where my bike was racked. I saw the camera crew waiting, asking, 'How do you feel?' For once words failed me. Steve managed to dodge them throughout, despite their interest in this mother/son duo. 'We'll get him in the morning when he goes to his bike,' they had told me, but he evaded them. I could see when Steve and I met up that he was just a tiny bit worried about me, which made me feel guilty. He had enough on his plate competing in an Ironman without having to worry about an ageing, mad mother.

The swim was fantastic. The stampede down the beach was of no concern to me: I am always happy to linger at the back and take my time rather than face the washing machine of two thousand athletes all swimming in a very small piece of water. Somehow, I found my rhythm and the few other slowcoaches who were swimming at my pace – mainly doing breaststroke. It was weird swimming over scuba divers with cameras. Canoeists were at the ready all the way and, despite my fear of water, it felt very safe, with opportunities to stop and hang on to the buoys, and the beach never more than four hundred metres away. I just loved the fish, some lovely and colourful, as well as tiny silvery blue ones in shoals. 'You are in a race,' I kept having to tell myself, 'this isn't a snorkelling expedition to see the marine life.'

It was tough, though. As I finished the first loop, the majority of competitors were getting out of the water, having done their 3.8k. I, and a few others, had to run up onto the sand, around a post and back in to the water for a demor-alising and somewhat slower lap two. I was the last but one person out of the water after the second lap – a guy came out and then raced past me up the beach so I was the last. I was enjoying the sensation of having finished an Ironman swim – it was far, far too much to race him as well. After the swim, it was back to transition and the all too familiar sight of my bike being the last one standing, but everyone I passed was so encouraging: 'Go Eddie!'

The bike course was by now a familiar route: out along the main road, and then off to the hills. I loved it, even the climb up to Fire Mountain, and down towards Club La Santa. And not long after that, the real climbs begin. Just before this point, a motorbike with a pillion rider approached, and went past. Then, to my dismay, I heard them do a U-turn and come up behind me. It was the film crew. I smiled and said

'Hi,' and then posed beautifully for them as we went through a small village, palm trees on either side. I was down on my tri-bars, every bit the expert cyclist. But then I started the beginnings of climbing the hill towards Haría, and realised I was moving rapidly out of my comfort zone. 'That's enough, guys,' I wanted to shout, or a few expletives, but I realised that wouldn't sound too good on film. Fortunately, just as I was really beginning to struggle up the hill they peeled off, waved, and said they'd see me on the run.

The next stage is the relentless climbing up and up, and then an incredible fast downhill round the bends. On a closed road, without threat of oncoming traffic, even I could release the brakes and enjoy. But once through the village of Haría comes the hardest climb of the lot. Will I, won't I, have to get off and walk up the steep bit I knew so well? Then there was another descent and another climb with a wall on my left-hand side. Finally, coming to the end of the wall was the moment I had been waiting for all day – that fabulous view down over the volcanic rocks to the bluest of seas and the island of La Graciosa. That picture has been my screen saver for years. One day I will do the Travesía a Nado El Rio, the famous annual swim from the beach below over to La Graciosa.

And then after the turnabout at the top of the mountain, and another Manrique creation at Mirador del Rio, comes the greatest descent ever – 10k of fabulous riding, beautifully resurfaced roads and gentle bends, down past the vineyards. I was already longing for midnight when I could have a glass of wine.

Eventually, I rode back into Puerto del Carmen, transition and then it was off on the run. As I went out, almost the first person I saw was Steve, coming to his final turnaround before doing his last lap. His grin said it all: his mum was safely out of the swim and had even finished the bike. To see him made me so proud – despite the frustration of knowing he would be in the bar for several hours before I had even finished.

I remember little of that run. They are never easy, but the support of the local community was fantastic and became more enthusiastic later on into the evening. After the first slope, which felt more like a hill, I saw Laurence Harding, Serpentine's top time-triallist. He had long finished and, typically, was out to support the slower athletes. 'Great, well done,' he shouted as I started the run, 'your Kona place is in the bag.' If you come first in your age group you get the option to purchase a slot at the World Ironman Championships in Hawaii. I was on target. I was the only woman in my age group and now I knew I was going to finish. It was dark, but I had plenty of time. Steve had by now finished and had a drink, but he was there to support me at each turnaround and even a bit further out on the run route.

Finally off I went on to the final lap, high-fiving and thanking people for their patient support as I ran. Then out into the quiet part, round the turn point and over the timing mat, and I was on my way back. The noise level was building over the last five hundred metres down the final slope. 'You are an Ironman!' I heard from the animated commentator. I ran through the gantry and into the arms of Kenneth Gasque. It had taken me 15 hours and 52 minutes. And then I met Steve and Jane for my dreamed-of glass of wine. It was an incredible feeling to have completed an Ironman. All those hours and hours of training had been worth it. I was walking tall, albeit with that stiff Ironman walk I had seen before, when out supporting Steve.

I had no intention of taking up my Kona slot but I will never forget Laurence's face when I told him I wasn't going. 'How could you? We would all die for the opportunity and you are rejecting it.' That sense of letting so many people down must have left its mark, as the following year I decided I would have to do my second Ironman Lanzarote and see if I could qualify. I vowed to take the training a bit more seriously and really focus on the swimming. So I booked a place on Steve Trew and Dan Bullock's brilliant annual training camp at Cesenatico in Italy, which offered great opportunities for hard-core swim, bike and run training.

I asked Steve how he had come to set up the camp, and why. 'I organised my first warm-weather training camp in 1987 after I'd been competing at a good high level for four years. I'd been on a couple of training camps and thought, I can do that. Of course, the learning curve was somewhat steeper than I'd anticipated. My objectives then were to give everybody – whatever standard or age – a good experience of structured training and, very importantly, to enjoy the experience. So what has changed in thirty years? Absolutely nothing. Well, actually what has changed is the average age of the athletes coming on the camps. This year the average age was fifty-two years young, with five athletes over the age of seventy. I guess we're doing something right. We are very fortunate that almost all of our athletes are returnees from the past thirty years; they've enjoyed previous camps and want to keep experiencing them. However, that doesn't mean that everybody just turns up and does nothing; on the contrary the training is tough and there's a lot of it but the evenings are focused around the athletes and we hold semi-mocking awards presentations throughout the two weeks at camp to ensure that everyone is recognised, whether it's for a personal best time or for having a puncture and getting into dinner late. Bottom-line objective: improve, learn and enjoy.'

And what a fantastic week it was, with great people and long-standing friends who were there for some serious training – and a strong social element that was the key to making it fun. These people were an annual presence at the Hotel Beau Soleil, where Dante, a former professional cyclist, would take us out on guided tours of the area, pointing out the home and training terrain of Marco Pantani, the brilliant cyclist, who won the Tour de France in 1998. He had won the Giro in the same year, but a year later was done for doping, which was thought to have led to his drug use and subsequent death by drug overdose. The annual Gran Fondo Nove Colli is a local race, strongly associated with Pantani. I was convinced that the required amount of climbing – nearly four thousand metres over 200k – was way beyond my competence level, but encouraged by Steve Trew and friends on the training camp, I decided I would train harder on the bike and have a go a year or so later.

I left the training camp three days early and came home, grabbed my Ironman kit, and was off again to Lanzarote. By then, I had left Parents for Children and was an independent social worker, able to control my own time effectively, and fit in the training, races and travels. Life was good.

I didn't make as big a dent in my previous year's finish time as I had hoped, although the swim was better. Again I was the only person in my age group, so when I finished I qualified for Kona. That race would take place four months later – was that giving a sixty-seven-year-old body enough time to rest and recover? Especially when I wanted to squeeze in one small race beforehand.

This race was called Ocean Lava. Kenneth Gasque was running it, and it was a Half Ironman distance based on the Ironman swim and a killer bike course up Femés, a climb well over 20 per cent at one point. What a challenge. I had wanted to do it to support Kenneth and his family, for whom I have so much respect and I felt it would be ideal final training before Kona.

The ocean swim was lovely, and it was a joy to be able to finish after just one lap. There was a beautiful schooner anchored out at sea for the turnaround, with an enthusiastic greeting by the crew. Out on the bike, the nerves really set in as the Femés hill approached. I pondered these increased anxiety levels as a steep hill gets nearer. I'd ridden up Femés before, on a camp when there was nothing was at stake; I had ascended successfully whilst a friend got off and walked. But in this race, with the anxiety flowing, as I reached the steepest bit, that awful moment of decision hit: should I get off before I fall off? Decisions, decisions, and then, suddenly I had no choice and I was off the bike. I walked the hundred metres or so around the bend to the café at the top. I wasn't the only one walking, but it was not a good feeling.

The evening reception and awards ceremony was the best ever. Wine flowed and the food was wonderful. It felt as though everyone on the island was out to support Kenneth's new race in any way they could. The meal over, Kenneth took the stage, and laughingly called out a few race numbers, mine included. He asked us to stand up. Anticipating yet another complimentary reference to my age, I held my head high only to be told that our small but select group of individuals standing were the ones who had walked up Femés. I loved the teasing, but it made me determined to practise on the steeper parts of the Surrey Hills, like Whitedown Lane.

Finally, it was on to Kona. At the risk of sounding like a jaundiced old woman, I am still asking myself why I didn't enjoy Hawaii anything like as much as Lanzarote in 2009 and 2010. To a large extent, I think I went because I could and thought I should. I know all too well the benefits of the positive discrimination. As a woman at my age, Ironman Lanzarote had to create an additional older female category, with its own Hawaii slot. I know, I can hear you all: it isn't fair that I just had to finish in order to qualify, when brilliant younger athletes can only dream of coming first or second in their age group and gaining a Kona slot.

A brief resume of Ironman and Kona. During the Waikiki Swim Club awards banquet in Hawaii in 1977, a naval officer and his wife, John and Judy Collins, started talking about which athletes were fittest: swimmers, runners or cyclists. They discussed the possibility of merging the toughest of each sport's races on the island; the Waikki Roughwater Swim (2.4 miles), the Around-Oahu Bike Race (115 miles) and the Honolulu Marathon. On 18 February 1978, fifteen competitors raced the first-ever Ironman challenge. Twelve finished the race, with Gordon Haller, whom I was to meet later at Ironman Lanzarote, winning.

When Collins no longer wanted to direct the Ironman race it was Valerie Silk who took control and moved it to the Big Island of Hawaii. The event received huge attention, particularly when in 1982 a student called Julie Moss collapsed and crawled to the finish line. It put Ironman onto the map and into commercial consciousness. In 1990 Silk sold the race and the brand (then known as the Hawaii Triathlon Corporation) for $3 million.

Now known as the World Triathlon Corporation (WTC), the company has grown into a formidable for-profit corporation. In 2007, WTC expanded into producing Ironman events and launched Ironman 70.3, the Half Ironman races. In 2008, WTC was purchased by Providence Equity Securities for an undisclosed sum. In August 2015, a Chinese company, Wanda, purchased it from Providence for $650 million.

As I understood it, race organisers pay the WTC for the Kona slots that they then allocate to age-group winners. This allocation takes place within twenty-four hours of completing their Ironman. In what is termed a roll-down, if winners of their categories choose not to take up their Kona place, the places can be allocated to a younger age group, where demand is so much greater.

So, I had the place in Kona and could return to the UK to tell Laurence, who had been so disappointed I hadn't taken up my slot before. If I thought the five hundred euros for the entry fee, that I had to pay immediately, in cash, was expensive, it continued to become a very costly adventure. Taking a bike on a plane was the first massive expense – I paid as much for the bike carriage as I did for myself. Then, accommodation rates are hiked enormously for that period. The listed price of seven nights in one of the central hotels was fifteen hundred pounds, so Hils, my fellow RAAM rider, who had also qualified, and I settled for a cheaper hotel about a mile and a half out of town. On reflection, though, even at the extra cost it might be better to have arrived earlier to acclimatise, and to be down in the hub of activity. Hils had been able to go out to Hawaii earlier and see the more attractive, greener and less commercialised side of the Big Island and I wish I'd been there to do the same.

The build-up over the last two or three days was not without incident. For the first time in my life I lost my passport. Instructions to go to the nearest UK passport office proved impractical as that was many, many miles away back in Los Angeles. Would it be possible to board a plane without a passport? I took a taxi ride out to the airport, where staff indicated that it might not be straightforward, and offered no solution. With stress levels building, I was struggling to see a way forward on the passport front – it was undoubtedly an extremely disconcerting experience and an added pre-race pressure.

Forgetting such minor problems as my inability to leave the island to go home, I was in Hawaii to do an Ironman, to enjoy, to make last-minute recces, rest and carb load. Gratefully, I took the opportunity for an organised practice swim with the buoys in situ, canoeists on the water, first aid on hand. Kona is always a no-wetsuit swim as the water is so warm, so I was absolutely dreading it. But once in the water, I was reassured. It really was warm and it was true: I was more buoyant in the salt water. The marker buoys were large and visible, and we were to swim out parallel to the beaches and the road back to our flat. For the first time in my life, a swim had actually de-stressed me!

Directly preceding the race, the atmosphere downtown and in the surrounding roads was, unsurprisingly, tense and quiet. This huge, annual event brings megabucks into the local community – one well-known coffee house apparently makes enough money in that week to cover their rent for a year. I have never seen so many fit, toned bodies in my life, all looking stressed as, in preparation for the big day, they rode, ran or swam the courses, or posed for their sponsors. This was the mecca of triathlon; everyone had trained for months, if not years, for this momentous weekend. The standard was so high. I could only respect the skill, dedication and determination that so many had brought to the event. I felt completely out of my depth and that I didn't deserve to be in such elite company.

The pre-race pasta party was far from special: a mass buffet with very basic and cheap food. No alcohol, but we could live with that. The professionals and the corporate visitors were corralled into their own space, with security guards keeping out us mere competitors.

But the Ironman film we were shown on huge screens was brilliant. It featured the old and the disabled, the young and the stories of courage. Showing that Ironman is an attainable dream for everyone – though there was no mention of cost.

The bikes get safely racked the night before the race. I noted with my non-expert view that there were some incredibly valuable bikes there, and that my three-year-old Specialized with a granny gear might not be the best on the block. The nerves were really building. And far from being the only one in my age group, I had a lot of company. The American and Canadian women have a fantastic tradition of Ironman racing, and in triathlons in general. There are many phenomenal athletes of sixty-five plus, with fifteen of us in Kona that year. I knew I was facing awesome competition.

Race day dawned. You get up for an early quick breakfast in the dark, balancing the need for calorie input with the need for food to digest in time to feel okay for the swim, and to make those last crucial trips to the loo. Then down by bus to the race start, to check over my bike in transition.

Finally, down towards the beach and the jump from the jetty into the water. Positioning myself towards the back and the side of the pack, I was sure I must be the slowest swimmer in the field of hundreds. After treading water for what felt like hours, the klaxon sounded and we were off, the swimming easier and calmer than I had anticipated. There was none of the jostling or bashing experienced by those competitive bodies up front. I was determined to go at my own pace and enjoy it. I kept saying to myself: you are the lucky one, you have made it to Kona and you are alive.

Amazingly, I made it out to the turnaround point, past the multiplicity of cheering boat crews, past the surfers, some standing up and some lying down on their boards, and then all the way back towards the start. Only in the last 1k or so was I really aware that I was towards the end of the swimmers, and that the surfers had very few bodies left that they needed to follow or maybe keep that extra-watchful eye on. My abiding memory of that swim is two gorgeous

bronzed surfers lying face down on their surfboards to either
side of me, paddling parallel, clearly directing me. And my
frustration that while my bi-lateral breathing meant I could
see both smiling, encouraging, tanned and fit-looking guys,
I couldn't talk to either of them. It also took me far too long
to realise I could have avoided lifting my head in order to
sight accurately as they were surely going in a straight line.
Still, my swim time was a personal best. As I staggered out
of the water I stopped to thank them both as they cheered
their old woman out.

Facing into the wind, I was on the bike. There were
no steep hills here, just straight, straight road, a bend then
more straight road, and then the hill. Up and up and steadily up. All on the same main road, the Queen Ka'ahumanu
Highway. Unlike other events, there were very few spectators. It just didn't have that same level of community support
as Lanzarote, where the Ironman is foremost an island event
to celebrate. Finally I hit the top of the hill and the famous
turnaround. The wind is known by this time to strengthen
and to change directions, but if it did, I didn't notice. I just
remember sobbing halfway down that hill. I was in Kona
doing an Ironman. I was the lucky one. Was Phil up there
supporting? Was his legacy to be my fighting determination
to get to the end of the race and make the most of my life?

It is a bleak route. For anyone used to the majesty of volcanic lava in the National Park in Lanzarote, the lava fields
of Hawaii are not impressive. Food and drink were available
at regularly positioned aid stations. I knew that I had to carb-
load at the last aid station on Queen K Highway, to fuel up
for the marathon ahead so was horrified to find they had run
out of energy bars and even bananas – only yet more energy
drinks. So, without carbs loaded for the run as planned, I rode
towards the end of the bike route, to transition and out onto

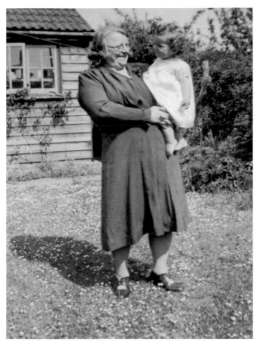

Proud grandmother, Georgina Landemare

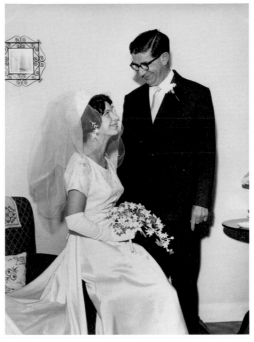

Loved my dad – my hero

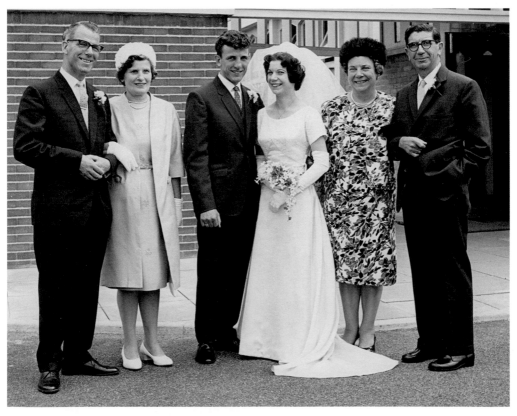

15 August 1964: my happiest day

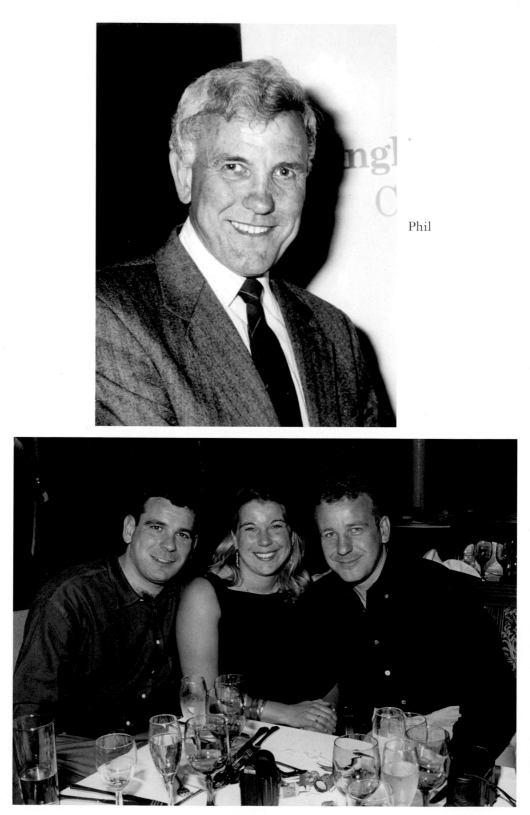

Phil

I love my kids

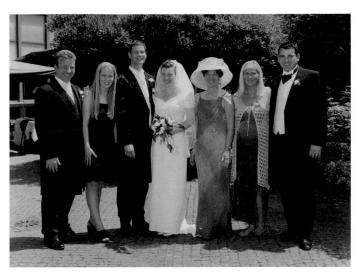

Family celebrations –
Kate and John's wedding

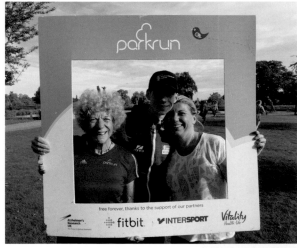

Intergenerational Parkrun
fun with Kate and Ben

Nottingham University,
22 December 2016

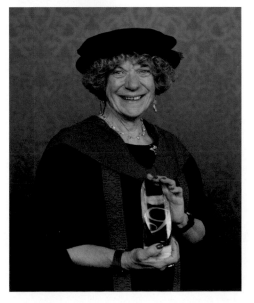

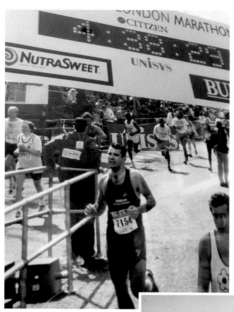

Gary finishing the London
Marathon – my goal

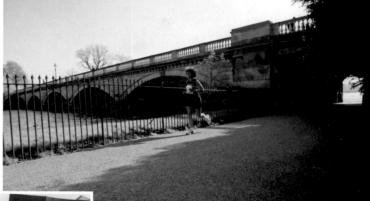

The Serpentine
Running Club
handicap race around
the Serpentine in
Hyde Park

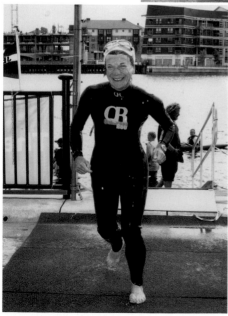

Best moment: the London
Triathlon swim done

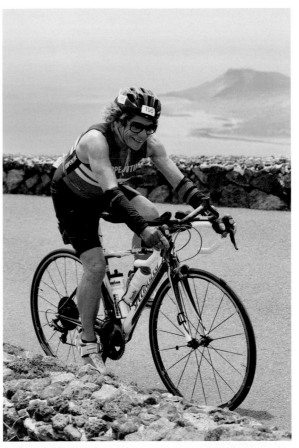

Ironman Lanzarote:
nearly at the top

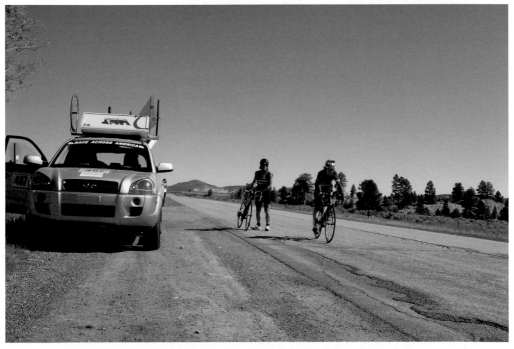

RAAM handover with Hils

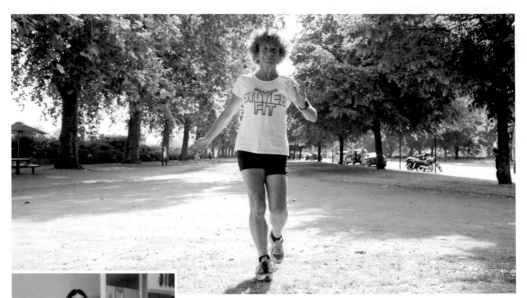

Photographed for the *Guardian* in Hyde Park

My friend, inspiration, Prosecco companion and coach Annie Emmerson

Silver cheerleading – always fun

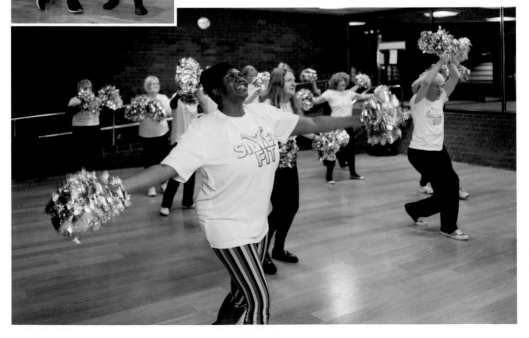

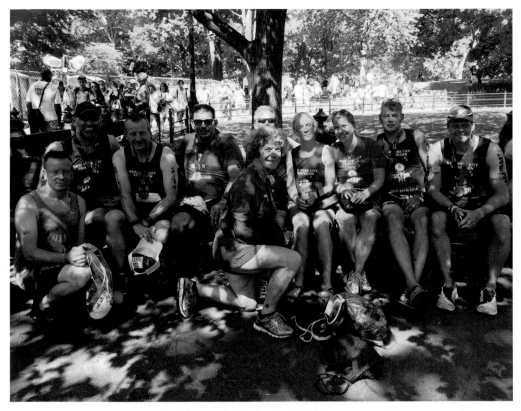

Family celebrations after the New York City Triathlon

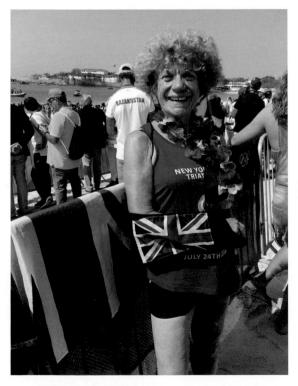

In Rio with my broken shoulder

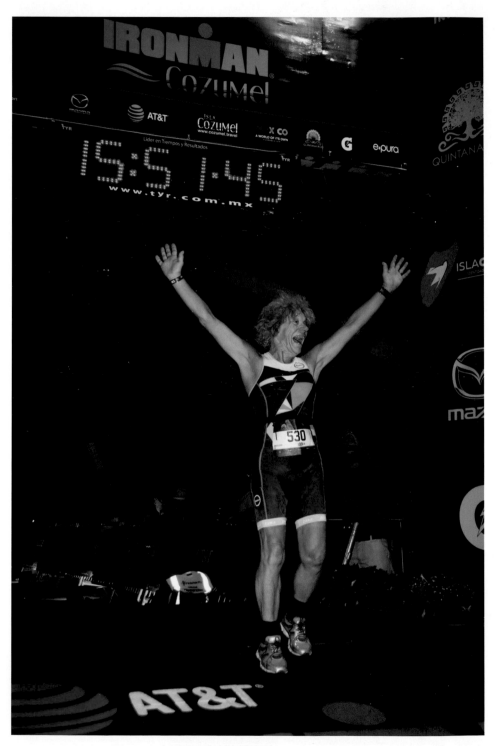

Irongran

the run. I was by no means the last – there were many cyclists behind me. Many were probably aware they were unlikely to make it back before midnight and the cut-off time.

With the sun beginning to drop, it was nothing like as hot for me as it had been for all those superb athletes ahead of me. There were a few miles in the town before heading out, again onto the Queen K. And my goodness how lonely that was. All the way out, for mile after mile before a turn to come back. The majority of the run route was along the same two-lane highway with just the occasional returning cyclist or race-related vehicle. There was a short, fun bit near the turnaround, with a big screen and some energising music. Then it was time for our head torches to go on.

The last 10k before hitting the town's boundary was unbelievably isolated. At this point, there were no runners coming in the opposite direction. We were all plodding along in the pitch dark on an empty motorway. By now, overtaking was rare. We were all at our limit. Coming into one of the final aid stations, there were a few minutes of respite and joy: lights, disco music you could hear a mile away, and, at last, the legendary chicken soup. It was great soup, but then back into that final dark, grim phase. How I missed the bars and fun of Lanzarote. The fact that I was in Kona was no compensation at all for the lack of friendly, supportive, good-humoured, often inebriated crowds along the run route. Certainly there was no evidence of a DJ on the course who would play Queen's 'Don't Stop Me Now' on request.

Then, finally, back into town and at last there were crowds to cheer you on for the last kilometre and into the finish area. As you approach the final metres you can see yourself coming over the line on the huge screen ahead, cameras ready to film you collecting your medal. An enthusiastic commentator shouted 'You are a sixty-seven-year-old social worker

Ironman!' My finish time was 15 hours, 41 minutes and 22 seconds. I was so pleased. After the medal was presented, two marshals guided me around and behind the screen, away from the lights, the crowds and the music. They pointed to the darkened area where my bag was, and then abandoned me.

I stooped stiffly down and picked my bag up, donned my jacket, and I was on my own – I asked a passer-by if there was any food and he pointed towards a tent a hundred metres away. There I was offered a slice of pizza, and was told, 'Sorry we have run out of ham, we only have cheese and tomato. Oh, and there is some ice-cream.' While ice-cream may be ideal for professionals completing the Ironman in the heat of the afternoon sun, it wasn't what I needed at 11 p.m. I asked if there was anything to drink and was pointed to another stand fifty metres away, offering energy drinks or water. That was Kona. I was so disillusioned. All this way. All that effort. All that money. All that razzmatazz, to be left alone with a slice of pizza and a container of energy drink.

Hils and I found each other and went out into the finish area to watch the last athletes come across the line and the heartbreaking sight at midnight of those whose path to completion was stopped by the Polynesian fire-eating ceremony. No mercy for all those athletes who hadn't made the cut-off.

Both starving hungry and alcohol-deprived, we knew we had to get our bikes out of transition within the hour. We walked slowly back along the main street towards our apartment, deciding to stop off for that first drink of wine at the same restaurant at which we had had dinner that first night. Our medals around our necks, we were greeted enthusiastically by everyone in the bar, but none so enthusiastic as one of the managers who came up to me: 'You were fantastic, I watched you come across the line – oh, and by the way I have your passport in a drawer in my office!' My relief was total. I remember very little of the rest of the night/morning as we celebrated.

That night the texts started to flow in. It was amazing how many people had followed the live feed, had watched my progress around the bike and run routes and seen me come across the line. My grandkids in Singapore and in London had seen me. That was impressive, but then I have never doubted the marketing reach of WTC.

And then the subject of the texts suddenly changed. From my coach Annie first: 'We've just seen you in *Spooks*!' Annie and her twin sister Charlotte had sat down to watch Iain Glen, Charlotte's partner, in the memorable BBC series about MI5 officers set in central London. They had seen the cameras pan down the Thames Path to follow an old runner ... me. Wow. I was a Kona finisher but, arguably much more significantly, I had been on *Spooks*.

8

Perception is everything

I am far from being a fit, injury-free oldie. But I continue to try. Indeed I have learnt so much from so many over the last twenty years, from pilates to yoga, coach to coach, and above all my brilliant and life-changing physio, Elaine Sawyerr from Belmont Physiotherapy. Crucially, she was the first person to identify the bunion on my right foot as a likely contributory factor to the muscle imbalance in my left leg.

At times, the professional advice I have been given has been conflicting – although my experiences may reflect fundamental professional approaches to injuries and ageing. By 2000, and with one serious disrupted ACL, I was recognising that I couldn't keep pounding the paved streets of London for ever. The wear and tear resulting from road running is an issue for most people over sixty.

Having become quite an expert on injuries and arthritis in the knee, and with pain around my medial ligament – one of the four major ligaments in the knee that runs down the inner part and connects the thigh bone with the shin bone – I was reminded of the song 'Dem Bones':

Toe bone connected to the foot bone
Foot bone connected to the heel bone
Heel bone connected to the ankle bone
Ankle bone connected to the shin bone
Shin bone connected to the knee bone
Knee bone connected to the thigh bone
Thigh bone connected to the hip bone
Hip bone connected to the back bone
Back bone connected to the shoulder bone
Shoulder bone connected to the neck bone
Neck bone connected to the head bone
Now hear the word of the Lord.

With these words in mind, I went to a physio who set me a three-week hard stretching programme for my calves and hamstrings. Despite all my efforts there was little change when I returned. It was the podiatrist who came into the room to offer a second opinion and saw my very high heels alongside the bed who realised why: 'Have you been wearing those? No wonder your muscles are still as tight. Try flatter shoes. Have you tried barefoot running, which strengthens the feet, both bones and muscles?'

A few months later, I had what I assumed was a bit of cystitis and I saw a locum GP who instantly prescribed some antibiotics without asking for a urine sample. When I returned with a slightly worse problem a week later, my own GP, clearly annoyed that the locum hadn't done a urine test, suggested I got up on the bed for examination. A bit of external prodding and poking and I watched his face fall. He had found a significantly sized lump that demanded pretty quick investigations.

For several days, test followed test and various instruments were inserted from below. I watched on the screen beside me as mini-bulldozers went into the wall of some part of my lower anatomy and suddenly grabbed a sample of me. Weird, but pain-free. I remember my controlled, outward calm, even though I knew cancer was the unmentioned word. Maybe because I didn't fully understand, or maybe because my husband had died and I had been the lucky one for an extra thirteen great years. I faced that possibility. But I could see that my daughter Kate, by now a senior registrar, understood far more than me. She came to all my appointments, and asked the questions I would never have thought of asking. She concealed her real fears from me, and only later did I learn from my sons how distressed she had been.

As on previous occasions, I reflected on the family dynamics of having a doctor in the house. How hard it is for a daughter and a younger sister playing so many roles with the extra layer of knowledge that can feel like power. After all the tests came the final out-patient appointment with Kate alongside me. I was gearing myself up emotionally to face the truth, only to be welcomed by an ebullient consultant. 'I have good news – you have a ruptured appendix, and we can remove that.' What a cause for celebration. The pink bubbly flowed for several days before I was admitted for surgery.

When the day came, I was sent down into a side room next to the operating theatre. I was the last patient for surgery that evening. The surgeon came into the room to speak to me briefly and I asked him, 'While I am under, is there any chance you could remove my hernia? I know I am sixty-five years old, but I can't wear a tri-top on the bike because the hernia sticks out.' It was only a small, longstanding lump below my chest, and it had never caused me any pain, but he laughed. When the anaesthetist greeted me, as they do just before putting you under, he too was laughing and said, 'I gather you want that hernia removed too.' Bless them, they did it. It is definitely the case in life that if you don't ask, you certainly don't get.

Following surgery, Steve and Jane were awaiting my return to the ward. Relieved that all was well, they left me. It was already late at night, but I can recall endless visits from the nursing staff all through the night. A junior nurse would check my heart rate and pulse, only to be followed minutes later by a more senior nurse to check the accuracy of her colleague's readings. I gather my fitness level meant my resting heart rate didn't fall within the normal range for my age.

The next evening Kate arrived for a visit and informed the nurses that she would take me out briefly in a wheelchair. I guess only a doctor would have been allowed to do that less than twenty-four hours after an appendectomy. Along the corridors, down the lift, we got to the hospital doors and there, across the road was Carluccio's. That glass of wine was irresistible. What fun. An hour or so later Kate wheeled me back into the hospital and quietly amidst all the sleeping patients, up on to the ward. I slept soundly and was awoken the following morning by the surgeon visiting his post-operative patient. 'I hear you went to Carluccio's last night. If you are that fit, you may as well go home today.' What a result! Recovery was swift and I was soon back to normal – further evidence of the fact that activity and strength training can promote faster recovery.

In 2011, I went back to Lanzarote to do the Ocean Lava triathlon for the second time, with two of the Serpentine Golden Girls RAAM team. My knees were a bit sore beforehand and I remember saying that if my left knee hurt I would run through it, but if the right knee (the one without an ACL) hurt, I would stop, all the time hearing my daughter over my shoulder: 'Mum, you are mad! Don't risk your knees – you are nearly seventy.'

I had completed the fabulous sea swim at Puerto del Carmen, and the tough, tough bike ride, including the iconic Fermés climb. And yet again I failed on that climb – but this year I was not alone: all of us were getting off to walk as the oncoming traffic was so congested. Relieved, I knew Kenneth Gasque could not make a laughing stock of so many of us again for having to walk. After the bike ride I went confidently out onto the run. In the event, my right knee didn't hurt, but on the second and final lap my left one suddenly started to hurt a lot. The paramedics were at the turnaround. I climbed into the nearby ambulance, where they bandaged it tightly and then suggested I ran on. I declined, saying that it wasn't that important for me to finish and that it was all about taking part. And anyway, I told myself, my left knee will recover really soon. I abandoned the race and had a ride back to base in the ambulance.

A month or so later, I was back having further MRI scans and going to see the orthopaedic surgeon. He spoke carefully, eyes on the screen in front of him, 'ACL deficient, arthritis level three to four.'

I replied, 'No, that's my right knee.'

'No, Eddie, it's your left.'

I was speechless: I hadn't heard the ping as that second ACL went, so how did it go? 'No one knows,' he told me, 'it can just happen, but there is no doubt: both your knees are now in serious trouble. Stop running now. Get out on the bike and enjoy pastures new.'

It was devastating news. I had loved running for nearly twenty years. Never the competing, just the running. Never the events, just the terrain – whether out in the countryside, along coastal paths, the hills and footpaths in the Peak District or along the Thames. The freedom, the smells, the flowers, the colour of the autumn leaves, the night lights of London. It was real grief and an absolutely massive sense of loss.

After reflecting for a week or two, I reasoned I could still do the Gran Fondo Nove Colli that I had promised myself two years earlier. It would be my new challenge; nine hills, 200k and 3840 metres of climbing – and being overtaken by 11,999 Lycra-clad cyclists. It could also be preceded by going to Steve Trew's Cesenatico camp for two weeks.

In preparation for the camp and the Nove Colli, I spent the spring on the turbo trainer, in spin classes or on rides in the Surrey Hills. I knew it would be a major challenge. I went to Cesenatico for the two weeks before the Nove Colli ride, and every day we went out, exploring some of those nine hills. There were also swim sessions every morning and evening with Dan Bullock, but I rejoiced that, as someone who couldn't run, I was no longer a triathlete and so didn't need to get up early and swim before breakfast. And even better, I could watch them all in the swimming pool in the evening, a glass of wine in hand. This is the life, I mused. I am a cyclist now, no longer a triathlete.

The hotel is about a hundred metres from the beach. On the way to a favoured beach bar is a lovely sandy path shaded by trees. It was here, six months after being told never to run again, that something made me put on some trainers and, for the first time, attempt to run again. I simply did a ten-metre jog followed by a forty-metre walk, then forty-metre jog and forty-metre walk and finally a long stretch of a hundred metres of relaxed running through the beautiful flat, sandy woodland stretch. I felt nothing in my knees and I was triumphant. Just maybe, I could run again. If I could run again, I might as well join a few of Dan's swim sessions too. Triathlon might yet be possible once more.

I popped down to the local beachwear shop, Karina's, and purchased the least flowery, least revealing one-piece suit I could find. It was a rather low-cut design but I figured, it was good enough for my slow pace of swimming. I didn't really think twice until the following night, when Dan was showing the whole group our individual swim sessions videoed earlier that day from an underwater camera in front of us as we swam down a lane. As he commented on individuals' technique, Dan was making suggestions for improvement. Suddenly it was my turn and there on the video was me, or rather my boobs – totally exposed. 'No, Dan. NO! Delete that video NOW! I don't want to know what's wrong with my catch, my rotation or even my pull in my freestyle swimming.' Dan still loses no opportunity to talk about that Karina video.

Re-energised by the odd run and swim, I joined the twelve thousand others on the fabulous Nove Colli ride later that week. The huge pelotons were scary. Twice I attempted to join them, only to be spewed out the back or the side, so I set-tled for riding at the side of the road, inevitably far, far slower, for 28k before the climbing began. Steadily, I climbed and descended the first three hills and then it was up Barbotto, where many were walking. But I had my eye clearly on my watch. I knew that, at the top of the climb, there was a cut-off at midday. If you didn't reach it in time, then you would be directed down the short route home. I climbed steadily up. It levelled off, another slight hill and there was the junction. The critical point of decision. Either it would be a sharp right turn and down towards the remaining five hills, or straight on, all the way down to Cesenatico, with no more climb-ing. But, I was telling myself, I wouldn't have completed the real race, the full nine hills of the famous Nove Colli. A race marshal greeted me and pointed firmly down towards Cesenatico as the cut-off time had now passed by several minutes. But close by were three or four police marshals. I looked plaintively at them and one of them shrugged his shoulders, and I am sure he pointed on to the full course of the Nove Colli. A quick right turn and down I went, fast, fearful that at any minute a race vehicle would come chasing after me. But I think they must have accepted that the mad, older woman had been very close to the cut-off time. Indeed, when I reached the drinks station a few kilometres further on there were loads of cyclists still there. I shot past without stopping, en route for hill number five, confident now that I was not the last and that the officials wouldn't come after me, the rhythm of 'Don't Stop Me Now' from a spectator's music system my driving force.

It is a hard ride. One of the toughest parts was a long, long downhill that led to pressure on all the joints that was new to me and came with no respite. I didn't dare move my hands away from the brakes. The other memorable experience was the short final hill, the steepest of the nine. But then the long beautiful views for the steady descent down to the coast. It was a lovely ride and as I finished at 11.30 p.m. I was well within the time limit. My risk-taking determination up at the top of Barbotto had been justified. A group from the camp was there at the end, waiting for me to finish. Later, the race dinner, a glass of wine in my hand and a band playing 'Don't Stop Me Now', was a wonderful celebration. What a fabulous day, or maybe it was thirty-six hours. Such is the joy experienced with many friends of all ages and all levels of skill and competence.

I came back from that Italian trip on a real high. Maybe, just maybe, I could run again. I sought a second opinion from Professor Fares Haddad, a leading orthopaedic and trauma surgeon at University College Hospitals, in June 2012. Armed with my scans of both knees, I was accompanied on this appointment by two of my children: Steve, the enthusiastic Ironman advocate, and Kate, the more cautious medical protector. Professor Haddad later wrote in a letter to my GP and copied to me:

She has bilateral longstanding ACL deficiency, she manages perfectly well although she has degenerative disease in both knees. She really came to discuss doing two Ironman triathlons. She has been advised to stop running, which was an eminently sensible decision but her motivation is such that she is desperately keen to get these two triathlons done. We have had a lengthy discussion today around the ways of reducing the impact on her knees by keeping them strong and doing most of her training away from running. She seems incredibly determined and is probably best guided in terms of her training and strengthening by a physiotherapist.

I tried one physio who immediately carried out ultrasound and told me that I would have to attend weekly. That I figured was likely to be a costly option. Fortunately, Prof Haddad had suggested a physio with a rather different approach. This was Elaine Sawyerr, who was not only concerned about treating my immediate symptoms, but also addressing the cause. This approach she said, would enable me to continue running whilst minimising further risk to my knees. Having determined that the underlying problem was my lack of muscle strength, she prescribed an extreme programme of strength and balance training and told me to return for a follow-up appointment only when I had completed it. I was immediately hooked by her clarity, her willingness to explain and interpret and her no-nonsense, practical approach. I am so, so grateful to Elaine for her enthusiastic, constructive advice over the past four years. She has given and continues to give me advice that is so relevant for older people and athletes negotiating the challenge of staying active while minimising the risk of injury and joint deterioration and damage.

Along with the ACL deficiency, I now understood more about my arthritis. I learnt there are over a hundred different forms of arthritis, the most common being what I have: osteoarthirtis, a degenerative joint disease. Elaine explained that she sought a balance between joint preservation on the one hand and bone health on the other. Load-bearing exercise, she emphasised, is recommended to maintain bone mass, particularly in women post-menopause who are at risk of developing osteoporosis. Load-bearing exercise has the potential to cause further joint damage, but crucially if done to minimise joint impact it has the beneficial effect of strengthening muscles and improving balance and proprioception, which are important components in maximising joint protection and injury prevention.

Achieving this delicate balance in my arthritic and ACL-deficient knee would enable me to continue to compete in triathlons whilst conserving my joints, which was my ultimate goal. I was hopeful for the first time that another triathlon might be within reach.

The basis of my rehabilitation programme was to enable me to exercise more efficiently, minimise impact loading on my knees and reducing injury risk in the longer term. In addition to the programme of strengthening and balance exercises for my lower legs and core, Elaine suggested I continue and perhaps even increase my training sessions on the bike and in the pool. The latter was low impact on my knees and would have the benefit of improving my overall muscle strength and endurance. She suggested that I run once a week, on an anti-gravity treadmill. This is a special treadmill that allows you to vary the amount of weight going through your legs, and was very helpful as it meant I could maintain my cardiovascular fitness whilst reducing the load through my knees. As my pain resolved and my knee strength increased, she suggested I add a 10k outdoor run once a week too.

Although I'm certainly not 100 per cent compliant, Elaine's programme enabled me to do what two years ago I would never have thought possible – to run, swim and bike without any pain. My running is at a slower pace, but even there Elaine challenged me. 'I don't understand why your running is slower – it shouldn't be.' Given how much progress I had made in strengthening my knee, which by now was pain-free, she could not see why my improvement was not translated into faster running times. Outside we went, so Elaine could watch me run up and down the road, only for her to tell me, in a very kind way, that my running technique was rubbish and that I didn't push off the front of the foot. Observing that my shoes could be the cause she suggested I go to a sports shop for an assessment to recommend more suitable shoes.

As I started to believe that I might just be able to get back into triathlon training, I began to do more research on government guidelines about combating the sedentary lifestyles of our ageing community.

Elaine shares my beliefs that physical activity offers one of the greatest opportunities to extend our years of active independent life, reduce the chances of disability and improve the quality of life for older people. Like me, she believes that the stereotypical perspectives of ageing, which encourage older people to 'take it easy', should be replaced with a more proactive model. A model that encourages older people to play a more active role in their own ageing. In my specific case, Elaine proposed a holistic programme that addressed my obvious injuries, but also minimised the risk of further injury and therefore would enable me to maintain an active lifestyle. She was, however, a little cautious about the new mantra 'exercise is medicine', cautioning that if people had specific problems they would benefit from specialist advice and treatment before starting exercise. This would limit the risk of injury progression.

In answer to my queries about how, despite arthritis, I was lucky enough not to experience any pain unless I was running downhill or making sideways movements, such as in step aerobics, Elaine explained that 'there is poor correlation between X-ray findings relating to osteoarthritis and the level of pain experienced. It is possible to have "bone on bone" (the most serious level) and no pain and conversely, one can have minimal joint changes and significant pain. The reasons for this disparity remain complex, but some of the modifiable factors relate to weight, strength, activity modification, co-existing injury, and advice.'

Elaine says that the key to maintaining an active lifestyle following a diagnosis of arthritis is initially to seek physio-therapy to determine and address the modifiable factors. If there is no success then seeking other specialist advice may be needed. This may include joint replacement surgery.

In discussing the need for variety in my programme, Elaine gave me the great image of a car made up of the chassis and the engine – the engine being the heart, the chassis being the skeletal system. While the engine would improve and become more powerful with cardiovascular exercise (walking, run-ning, etc), the chassis would be put at risk of breaking down if it wasn't strengthened to cope with the increased power being driven through the wheels. In a nutshell, she explained that strength training is equally as important as the activity you wish to perform in minimising injury risk and improv-ing performance. Strength training is particularly important to an ageing musculoskeletal system due to changes in joint mobility, stiffness, balance and muscle strength.

Elaine set me the following programme, which although individualised, contains some valuable suggestions for all us oldies.

Strengthening

My injury had caused significant weakness in my leg muscles but ageing may also have had an effect as it results in a loss of muscle mass. Elaine recommended:

- Weight training for lower leg muscles (quads, hamstrings, adductors, abductors, calves)
- Strengthening of the core muscles three times a week
- The use of a muscle stimulator for the quadriceps to address the muscle timing and balance issues between the vastus medialis obliqus (VMO) and the vastus lateralis (VL)
- A BodyPump class once a week. At my first class I was far too ambitious, using weights that were much too heavy for a novice. I could hardly move my shoulders for days afterwards and have to admit I've tended to shy away since

Cardiovascular fitness and endurance

I was encouraged to continue running using an anti-gravity treadmill, swimming and cycling, but with a greater emphasis on shorter runs and longer bike and swim sessions.

Flexibility

I was given a programme of stretches for the major leg muscles (quads, hamstrings, calves). The issue with stretching is usually that very few do it enough.

Balance and coordination

Elaine said she had noted a reduction in my single leg
balance that could be the result of my deficient ACL and/
or age which has an effect on sensory input and motor
activity. The ACL has an important function in providing
sensory input to the brain, which modulates muscle activity around the knee and balance. I was given a programme
that included balance exercises using wobble and balance
boards, and exercises on one leg.

I reassured myself that I was feeling fit and I was looking
forward to the triathlon season ahead. I rarely watched TV,
and did fifteen to eighteen hours' training each week, so I
certainly couldn't be described as having a sedentary lifestyle.
Unexpectedly, I started to experience a bit of back pain and
other minor symptoms. A visit to the GP led to yet more
intrusive camera work, numerous blood tests and scans. I
had an extremely anxious ten days leading up to Christmas.
Coinciding as it did with the twenty-year anniversary of Phil's
death, it was a tough time for all of us. Finally, on Christmas
Eve, the fantastic NHS consultant at Guy's Hospital confirmed
that all was okay on the big–C front. Kate and I celebrated at
the top of the nearby Shard before going on to our favourite
annual BT Christmas concert at the Albert Hall.

But I began to reflect that maybe I was pushing an older
body into too much training.

Yet again it was Elaine who asked the right question about
my intermittent back pain. 'How long do you spend at the
computer?' I responded that I could manage five hours at a
sitting. Elaine gasped and told me that thirty minutes is the
absolute limit, after which we should all get up and move.
She advised that my pain was coming from the fifth lumbar
vertebra and the surrounding tissues, through which most

of one's upper body weight is transmitted when sitting. Our sedentary jobs and way of life make us all vulnerable to this type of problem. Too much time in front of the television or computer, not enough exercise and poor posture can cause subtle strain in the skeletal system that may lead to injury over time. Elaine suggested I remedy the problem with specific exercises for my lower back, and more swimming.

Swimming is a low impact way of exercising and is easier on your joints than other sports such as running or cycling. As the water can support up to 90 per cent of the body's weight, I know swimming is good for those with disabilities, injuries or illnesses like arthritis. Additionally, swimming offers a unique feel-good factor that only being in water offers, long before the endorphins or 'runner's high' kicks in. Somehow, despite my relative dislike of swimming, I always get a great relaxed feeling afterwards, even just I've just done a few lengths. One day, when I am no longer able to run, and maybe even bike, I just hope I will be able to spend five minutes in a swimming pool. Sometimes, as I go for a spin session at 7.25 a.m., there are groups of older people leaving the sports centre after their early-morning swim. Impressive, and I am sure the ideal wake-up call.

I still often wonder how I will cope if I do have to withdraw from exercise. My fifty years of social work and my research have led me to explore some of the more driven personalities. I recognise many of my traits there and accept that I am always looking for the next goal and feel lost without one. Clearly it is a form of addiction. With exercise addiction estimated to affect up to 5 per cent of runners we can feel physical and emotional withdrawals in the absence of exercise, like those addicted to other substances. And I dread the day when I really, really won't be able to run or bike.

So how do others cope with the withdrawal of exercise and sport, due to injury or the ageing process? I have met and read about quite a few exercise junkies or top sports people who have reached retirement with varying degrees of success. What enables some to cope, adjust and, crucially, find other challenges? Everyone has some periods of feeling low or depressed, but while some divert their goal-driven energies effectively, others sink into other addictive behaviours or longer periods of mental distress.

Steve Trew commented that 'coping with age, injury and withdrawal symptoms is very real to me. My entire life has been sport; taking part, teaching, coaching, writing, commentating and watching. When I was competing and training, it felt very strange if I had to miss a training session, it was something that I *had* to do. Aches, injuries, minor illnesses notwithstanding, I needed to train; it was part of me, what I did, who I was. But as with most athletes, injuries and age and (particularly) over-use injuries came more and more to the fore. For me, triathlon was an absolute blessing. It meant that I was able to train at least twice a day without suffering the injuries and aches from running twice a day. But 'even Radio Caroline died' (showing my age now) or, in my case, my knees finally said "no more". Six years on from a new titanium knee and at the grand old age of seventy years young, I'm happy that I can *still* train at least once a day; my lovely, lovely swimming all my life and lovely cycling, which – if it hasn't quite taken the place of running – is a pretty good substitute.'

My coach Annie Emmerson is a wonderful example of coping with retirement after being a professional athlete – and world duathlon champion. Starting with coaching, she has then focused her energies into motherhood and TV commentary. In nine years of friendship, I have never seen that feeling of despair. She is still fit and, at forty-five, able to do a marathon in fractionally over three hours and an eight-mile run in under fifty-five minutes. Annie was clearly at the extreme end of the skilled athletic activity spectrum. Others, like some of the footballers we know only too well from the media, have made far less successful transitions away from their celebrity-athlete status.

Two friends from Serpentine Running Club have had their sporting lives taken away from them through adversities we would not want to imagine and I have learned so much from their inspirational stories.

Jan had competed in many sporting events over the years gaining medals along the way. She had completed a few ultra-marathons, including the London to Brighton and the Comrades Marathon in South Africa, and had won silver and bronze medals in the World Age-Group Duathlon Championships. However, in late 2011 she contracted meningitis as well as septic arthritis, which left her incapacitated. After the acute illness was over, Jan had to learn how to walk again. Originally hospitalised in December 2011, she was finally released in February 2012, by which time she had graduated from a wheelchair to crutches. After seven months she was able to progress to one crutch and finally three months later she left that crutch at home too.

Asked what kept her motivated through such an awful period, Jan said that as she was used to following training regimes before her illness, she believed in exercise programmes delivering results. She spoke too of the network of family and friends that had always kept her motivated. She reflected that training partners and running club friends were enormously supportive, with visits and messages while she was in hospital. Once she was home, they offered practical help with some of her exercise programmes and with getting around. The hospital physios in neural rehabilitation had provided daily guidance and support, with weekly goal-setting and reviews. In addition NHS physios, and a private physio who has treated her for ten years, were invaluable. She felt that the most rewarding aspects of fitness were the friendships she had developed on conversational runs and the support of training partners. 'There's a feel-good factor that comes with exercising and I have been able to go and see sunrises with dawn runs in some amazing places.'

Jan had been motivated too by Kate Allatt's book *Running Free: Breaking Out from Locked-in Syndrome*. A fun-loving mother-of-three, Kate Allatt's life was torn apart in her thirties when what had seemed to be a stress-related headache exploded into a massive brainstem stroke, leading to locked-in syndrome. Totally paralysed, she became a prisoner inside her own body. Doctors warned her family she would never walk, talk, swallow or lead a normal life again. But they didn't know Kate. The words 'no' and 'never' were not in her vocabulary. With the help of her family and best friends she drew on every ounce of her runner's stamina and determination to make a recovery that amazed medical experts. Using a letter chart, Kate blinked the words 'I will walk again'. Soon, she was moving her thumb and communicating with the world via Facebook. Eight months after her stroke, Kate said goodbye to her nurses and walked out of hospital, to return home and learn how to run again.

With similar resilience, Jan has shown us all, with remarkable courage, how she has moved on to acquire new skills. She joined the Serpentine Swimming Club and went on to be part of their seven-woman relay team that swam the Channel in 2015. I was lost in admiration of the group, training in the Serpentine, then down in Dover and finally the real Channel crossing — and all without wetsuits!

Jan is currently doing some ten-mile cycle time trials, and although she says she is the slowest competitor in the field she adds: 'That doesn't matter, because you are really racing against yourself. But you're also out there mixing it and feeling part of the action, with heart rate at race level. And, to keep myself out of mischief and have a bigger goal, I am also training for Coniston Water in September. This swim is the length of the lake – 5.25 miles – and for me will take as long or longer than running a marathon used to.'

My own minor injuries and health problems clearly pale into insignificance compared with Jan's, and also the injury recovery and driving force of Manuel Moreno.

Manuel said he had always been reasonably fit and used to play football at school. As he grew up, he enjoyed walking in the countryside, but he also smoked and drank 'a bit'. At fifty years of age, he decided to stop smoking. He started to run and joined Serpentine Running Club, and increased the distances.

Then, when he was sixty-nine, Manuel had a terrible accident. Cycling back home from his local Sainsbury's in Ladbroke Grove, he was hit by a lorry. His right leg was crushed, and subsequently had to be amputated just below the knee. He was wheelchair-bound, initially being pushed. Manuel's recovery was supported by the physio department of St Mary's Hospital, where he met many servicemen with similar, horrific injuries. But three years later, despite the amazing help he got from the prosthetists, walking remained difficult and painful, and he still could not run. Mentally, he was finding the adjustment very difficult.

As a longstanding friend, Manuel knew of the Silverfit sessions we had started in Hyde Park, where he was helped by the instructor to get back on a bike, with the necessary adaptations, and he now says, 'The bike was my salvation. I

found a way with some support, companionships and friendship of Clarion Cycle Club. It's belonging, feeling vulnerable
and humble yet it's possible. It's one pedal at a time, one rotation, one revolution.' He cycles on the roads of his London,
and with friends rode an incredible one thousand miles from
London to Barcelona, averaging 100k every day for sixteen
days, without a rest day and in serious heat between 32 and
38° Celsius. He says they'd stop for lunch, including wine
and beer, and always a beer before the end of the day's ride.
They planned to enter Spain at Le Pertus, like their Clarion
Cycle comrades had done in 1936/7 to defend the republic
against Franco's forces.

The team of eight riders made it in July 2017, having gone
through one town at the same time as the Tour de France, and
even making the news on the same page of the local paper.

Both Manuel and Jan had a basic underlying fitness from
their earlier running history, and mental courage to move on.
But both emphasised the importance of their social networks,
their friends and colleagues in the Serpentine Running Club.

How, then, can we help others facing similar crises, or
just the process of ageing, if they haven't had the benefits
of such a background? My awareness of the mental strength
I had gained from being 'the lucky one' has without doubt
influenced my determination to enable Silverfit to access and
then help those oldies who lack the athletic backgrounds of
Jan, Manuel and myself. For the three of us, that essential
sandwich recipe of social, physical activity and more social
has proved invaluable.

9

Take every opportunity
to inspire others

As I started my transition from social work to the fun of taking part in running and triathlon events, the sporting side of my life was all low-key in media terms and I had absolutely no desire for any personal publicity. After all, I was a social worker and confidentiality was vital. I remember my embarrassment when leaving the family home of a man who was to feature in a high-profile case and being caught on camera, and the image then appearing on the front page of a newspaper. I could never, ever have predicted the difference just a few years would make in terms of the media interest in an old woman doing Ironman and setting up Silverfit.

So, what drives me, and why? How much of my energy is down to genes or my life experiences I leave others to decide. But far more importantly, retirement after my fifty years in a wide variety of social work has left me with a sense of fulfilment and satisfaction in a job as well done as I could manage. I only finished my role as a consultant linked with court proceedings when I felt I needed to devote more time than I had available to ensuring my legal and policy knowledge remained up to date, and that I could do the families and their children justice. My high energy level was clearly linked to my ongoing enthusiasm, level of activity and an increasing interest in promoting healthy ageing and supporting the government guidelines to 'Get Active, Every Day'. What could I do to help build a fitter, happier, older generation, able to enjoy life as much as I was and gaining new friends as I have done through sport?

To raise funds for the adoption agency Parents for Children back in 2007, we organised some trail marathons in the beautiful Lee Valley. The route came down to what was to become the Olympic Park. Every year we watched the venues develop, particularly Lee Valley Watersports Centre, the Aquatics Centre and the velodrome. The first trail marathon, in 2007, was called Five2Go, then it was Four2Go, Three2Go, Two2Go, and finally One2Go in 2011.

We learned some hard lessons as event organisers – a short marathon distance in Five2Go and poor route signage two years later had both led to complaints – but by One2go it was all working perfectly. We also organised a family festival on Hackney Marshes, with intergeneration relays and a 5k. There was even a race for black-cab drivers – who, we realised, could lead remarkably sedentary lives.

After Three2Go, I left Parents for Children, which had by then been merged with a larger adoption and fostering agency, to return to my role as a social worker and independent expert witness. Together with some Serpentine Running Club friends and fellow athletes we set up a separate charity called Sporting Bunnies and continued to run the trail marathon events down the Lee Valley and were so proud to be awarded the INSPIRE mark. Two of the four stated aims of the Olympic Legacy had been to promote community engagement and to encourage the whole population to be more physically active. The London 2012 INSPIRE programme was established to 'recognise outstanding non-commercial projects genuinely inspired by London 2012 Games', as an agency associated with the legacy of the 2012 Olympic Games in London. The pink INSPIRE logo was to act as a promotional tool to reach out to new audiences. I think we have done, and continue to do it justice.

From 2006, I had been participating in the Parkrun at Bushy Park in south-west London – I have an unusually low Parkrun registration number of 596. Parkrun is the absolutely brilliant concept of Paul Sinton-Hewitt and his team of volunteers, offering a free timed 5k run every Saturday morning. It started out as the Bushy Park Time Trial in 2004, and is now in an incredible 460 venues worldwide. I helped to set up the Hackney Marshes Parkrun, building on our 5k route of Two2Go and risk assessment.

After One2Go we resolved in Sporting Bunnies to have a year off and enjoy the London 2012 Olympics and Paralympics. I loved the whole experience. I had managed to get four tickets for the hockey and was able to exchange them for two at the velodrome. I am ashamed to add that yet again, I didn't make enough allowance for the crowds, and the distance from Stratford station to the velodrome – I'm sure very few people who had a full morning's ticket managed to miss Chris Hoy in his 9.00 a.m. event. I did get to see many of the free events such as the cycling road race and the triathlon. Best of all was the thrill of watching Bradley Wiggins on the final four hundred metres of his cycling time trial. You knew he was approaching from Bushy Park as the noise of the crowd beating the hoardings that held us back from the cyclists hit a crescendo as he passed. He took the widest line of any of the competitors as he swept round that final corner to Olympic gold, and then sat, memorably, on that gold throne outside Hampton Court Palace.

We had a great day in the stadium for the Paralympics, with Steve Trew commentating and David Weir and Hannah Cockcroft performing so brilliantly. And then the most expensive but utterly memorable experience of the closing ceremony of the Paralympics. What an incredible spectacle, not to mention Coldplay, Rihanna and Jay-Z. It was so moving to watch all the war heroes and so, so many other athletes who were, despite their disabilities, getting so much from sport and teamwork. The swirling neon lights that engulfed the stadium were incredible, each seat glowing in pinks, oranges, yellows, greens and blues. The fireworks display and the torch finally extinguished. It was an incredible six weeks.

Everyone had enjoyed 2012 so much. That made a few of us oldies reflect: how could we follow it, contribute to the legacy and make a difference? How could we promote healthy ageing to an increasingly inactive and isolated older generation? It probably wasn't, we concluded, by organising more trail marathons, which after all were aimed at people who were already fit and active.

So along with our longstanding volunteers, many of whom were older Serpentine Running Club members, Gamesmakers and good friends, we had a brilliant brainstorming meeting asking ourselves how we could make a difference to the future. We knew the theory; we knew the overwhelming research evidence of the benefits of a healthy lifestyle, taking on board the magic formula of good nutrition, no smoking and regular exercise, along with a good social network and only moderate alcohol consumption. Given the dramatic emergence of the obesity epidemic, the rise in type 2 diabetes and sedentary lifestyles, it is similarly clear that the risks and costs are higher for the over-fifties, both for the individual and for society with the younger generation forced to pay the health and social costs of dependent elders.

We also recognised the powerful commercial and political influences opposing living a healthier lifestyle. The power and marketing budgets of the junk food industry, the drinks industry and the meat industry are huge and appear to influence overall media coverage. We questioned why companies like Coca-Cola were able to link their name with opportunities to be more physically active. 'Get out into local Parks, be less obese,' Coca-Cola suggested, while selling sugar-filled drinks.

Moreover, a costly focus on screening, rather than prevention, for things like cholesterol and blood pressure results in a 'solution' via the pharmaceutical industry. Pills do not tackle the underlying causes of type 2 diabetes. We knew that greater funding for prevention and working out ways to overcome the blocks to a healthier lifestyle could be far more advantageous. Attempts by doctors to prescribe exercise via programmes in gyms has not been wholly successful, in terms of both take-up and maintenance.

We felt the Olympic legacy offered a platform for motivation, inspiration, media coverage and a new range of realistic goals for the over-fifties. And we knew that INSPIRE 2012 would be considering the legacy for older people. We believed that with partners such the Olympic legacy, the Mayor's office and GLL/BETTER, and with the support of other charities, corporates and statutory agencies, we could find more fun, sociable ways to motivate permanent change in lifestyles.

The least active members of our population are also the least fit, happy and healthy. There are undeniable social determinants of healthy ageing. Poverty plays a massive role. So, if we were aiming for 'successful ageing and quality of life', then we needed to find ways of overcoming these blocks, and fitter over-fifties need to demonstrate the way forward, and to motivate others to do the same. We knew that offering individual counselling, enabling fitness tests and measuring goals in GP practices has been proven to be effective. And we saw the difference that volunteering at events and activities had also made to encourage those fifty-year-olds to get fitter and feel fulfilled.

We had registered as a charity to run the 2Go events, so by February 2013, were able to change our name. We took our focus into account, and came up with the name Silverfit. Immediately we realised how appropriate it was – Silverfit would 'do what it says on the tin'. One of our colleagues designed a logo and another Serpentine runner trademarked it on our behalf. As a charity, we reviewed our aims and objectives, secured funding from Sport England and set up our first Silverfit Silver Tuesday sessions in Hyde Park by August 2013. Could we build up steadily, find out what worked and what didn't? Could we, as a charity uniquely, we thought, run by older people for older people, create our own oldies' formula to scale up and get the message out there that it was never too late to get a bit more active?

Silver Tuesdays offered a range of physical activities to encourage the development of new, more active social networks. With the support of Sport England, we created Silver Tuesday sessions in Burgess Park in Southwark, then several other London venues, and then expanded to cover every weekday. By early 2017, there were eighteen venues up and running, with more in the pipeline.

With our unique sandwich formula – a Silverfit session comprises socialising, then physical activity, followed by more socialising – we explored a range of different activities, all with varying benefits for mind and body.

Nordic walking is one of the most popular outdoor Silverfit activities. It is a full-body exercise that suits people of all ages and fitness levels, providing health benefits for everyone – from those with medical conditions to the super fit. Walking with poles is great for increasing core stability, and facilitating balance. It is a sociable activity too, with all the benefits of being outdoors in some fabulous parks and woodlands as the seasons change.

Pilates is also very popular. Brigit helped us as our first pilates instructor, and she also gave us key marketing advice at the beginning. Bogusha, another of our instructors, is also a physiotherapist and says that pilates principles have complemented her professional experiences, giving her pain-free freedom of movement. She is an advocate for re-aligning, re-balancing, re-centring – just to list a few of Pilates principles – to enhance the performance, reduce the occurrence or alleviate existing injuries by creating awareness and utilising core muscles, which take the strain from the joints.

Silver cheerleading and Latin American dance. I met Zoe Rutherford, the director of the London Cheerleaders, at a public health conference and I went with her to Twickenham to watch her team cheerleading at a rugby match. Together we immediately saw the potential for silver cheerleading. Zoe sent me a great BBC film of Japanese older women cheerleading, and that was the beginning. It is a fun activity for men as well as women, with great music and non-gymnastic moves, which along with the warm-up routine helps to improve balance and core strength. Above all, there is a smile on everyone's face. Evidence shows that activities which include multiple components improve cognitive functioning to a greater extent than simple aerobic exercise. A six-month trial found dancing had beneficial effects on attention, reaction time, subjective wellbeing and posture, hence the popularity of our Latin dance sessions in one venue.

Walking football was created in 2011 to help keep players involved in football for longer. Games are played at a slower pace, in theory to reduce the threat of pain, discomfort and injury. If a player runs then they concede a free kick to the other side. This restriction, together with a ban on slide tackling, is aimed both at avoiding injuries and at enabling those who would not be able to cope with the real game to play football again. From many observations, though, I know a firm referee is required to ensure participants are walking not running, and that the ball is kept below head height. The size of the pitch can vary to suit different locations. Whilst it does promote cardiovascular fitness and helps participants maintain an active lifestyle, it offers a crucial social outlet with a purpose that may tempt those more socially isolated to get moving again and have fun in a sport they have loved all their life. Most of us first saw it featured in the Barclays Bank advert in 2014. Silverfit has worked with Millwall FC, Crystal Palace, Fulham and the London FA to develop our weekly sessions with our mixed teams. Walking football for women is beginning to take off too. Sadly us oldies had no experience of playing football when we were younger, so tackling is a new concept.

Bollywood fitness is another popular activity. It is based on Bollywood dance including Bhangra, a Punjabi folk dance. But our charismatic leader, Tamanna, has used the energising music and adapted some of the dance movements to offer a gentle all-body workout. A smile on everyone's face is guaranteed and it accommodates a range of physical abilities, with several eighty-plus-year-olds moving to the rhythm of Bollywood music. We love the exercises with tassels and pompoms, and even a large parachute to dance beneath.

Spinning. I have loved and benefited hugely from spin biking over many years. However tired I am when I arrive, it never fails to energise me. It relieves all the stresses, and the pounding music ensures I pedal at a rate that burns calories and builds muscle tone at the same time. Turning the dial increases the bike's resistance and works those muscles. Pedalling faster burns the fat. Above all, sessions are fun and can be as easy or hard as you choose, which makes it ideal for the range of fitness within Silverfit. Again, for me it is the music that makes the difference, and inspires me to increase the cadence just that bid more. The reggae music at Brixton is my favourite or maybe Queen and 'Don't Stop Me Now'!

Qigong and tai chi. One of our tutors, Sareera, insists that the benefits of Yang-style Qigong and tai chi for those forty-five-plus are incredible, as a low-impact and relaxing form of exercise. Tai chi and Qigong are the internal Chinese martial art in the sense that they focus on mental and spiritual aspects integrated into movement. She uses a meditative form of Qigong exercise at the beginning, followed by a dynamic tai chi spear form and ends with a meditative series of movement. All the Silverfitters report on the relief of stress and mastering the deep breathing techniques, and easing of arthritis pain and crucially the improvement of balance and stability. Research indicates that it promotes faster recovery from strokes and heart attacks as well as improving the onset or deterioration of dementia. The laughter around the routines with those colourful fans clicking open and closed is notable.

Yoga is a fabulous exercise for all ages, but most specifically as we age. As Colette O'Neill, a yoga therapist and triathlete, wrote, the body is as young as the spine is flexible. As flexibility decreases with age, particularly the spine, yoga can counteract this with low-impact exercise, providing strength training using body weight rather than added weights, reducing the risk of injury. Specific poses can improve balance to protect against falls and helps to protect joints, and promote bone health. Practising yoga relaxation techniques for thirty minutes has immediate beneficial effects on brain function and performance. As with other group classes they provide a social and fun environment, and in a golden thread running through all Silverfit activities, it is the social interaction too that reduces the risk of depression, anxiety and isolation.

Regenerative walking. After a couple of Silverfit regenerative walking sessions with Alex Swainson I learned to adapt my walking style. Alex has developed a seven-step walking method, which includes working with gravity, shortening the stride, leading with the hips and relaxing the jaw and core. He suggests we use the natural weight of our arms, imagining our hands are made of lead, to generate and and sustain movement like a pendulum. I find myself, despite the shortened stride, to be faster, and it has been of massive benefit when I resort to walking as part of the 'run' component of a triathlon.

Badminton is a sport combining all kinds of physical fitness. Although I had never been able to connect the racquet with the shuttlecock myself, I had spent so many hours watching Gary and all the junior players, and I loved the dynamics, akin to playing chess. Like other sports, it provides all-round exercise that helps us to live a longer, healthier life. But although it can be a fast-paced game, improving speed, it is sociable and an ideal indoor option. Silverfit is helped enormously in Haringey by having Clasford Stirling as our instructor. As a community youth worker running the community centre on the troubled estate of Broadwater Farm that has seen the riots of 1985 and 2011, Clasford was awarded an MBE for his work. He has used physical activity, and football in particular, as a way of engaging the youth and reducing the crime rate. It is such a privilege to have him on board helping the local older generation get more active too!

Within Silverfit we have also had the privilege of organising a series of sunset aquathlons in Hyde Park every summer. After a 500-metre swim in the Serpentine, participants go for a 5k run in Hyde Park. Race-directed by Runrite, Silverfit provides all the marshals and it proves to be a fun opportunity, as well as a fundraising source.

Alongside the weekly Silverfit sessions, we knew we needed to campaign and spread the message about the importance of activity and socialising for the over-fifties. It is a core aim of the Silverfit charity. Susie Symes, a friend and fellow Serpentine member, suggested that I write a piece for the *Guardian* Running Blog about my training programme for Ironman Lanzarote in 2013. Susie was sure I must be one of the oldest, if not *the* oldest, women in the UK to do an Ironman, and thought it would be of interest. But I was plagued by doubts. Would I be able to finish the Ironman? Would my knees still stand up to it? What a fool I would feel if I had publically talked about it and then failed dismally, even though I could understand that such a failure might be motivating. In the end, I took the cowardly path of waiting until I had done the Ironman before writing my first post later that year.

I put that blog up on the *Guardian* website late one night and I was amazed when, first thing the next morning, one of their journalists was on the phone. They wanted to feature my story in their review section and would be sending a photographer out that same day. For the first time, I appreciated the significance of what a PR company had once told me of the importance of the ST factor: fastest, oldest, slowest, happiest. The ST factor commands attention. I realise I will never be the fastest and sometimes I maybe the slowest but I know I am usually the oldest and if that makes a great story to promote Silverfit then I will be the happiest. And the photo the *Guardian* took of me jogging down the tree-lined avenue in Hyde Park remains one of my favourites.

I was totally unprepared for the publicity that followed. I have now been in most newspapers, on TV far too much and had some offers to be on gameshows, though I drew the line at doing those. I've even made it onto a Tube poster. I agreed to be one of the three 'living legends' for Remember a Charity, a campaign to persuade people to leave money in their will to a charity of their choice. Cheerfully, I gave my time for photoshoots and filming, never ever dreaming my image would be used in those huge posters in Underground stations. Seeing a massive picture of myself as a living legend, gazing down on the Tube platform was amazing but disconcerting.

Deep in Stockwell station, I took my first selfie of the poster. Proudly I sent it to Ben, my grandson, who had set me up as Madgranny71 on Instagram. He came back patronisingly: 'Well done Eddie, you've done your first selfie.' Less than a minute later the penny obviously dropped, and a second message followed: 'OMG'.

I am not someone who relishes the public eye but over the years have been persuaded by friends and the trustees of Silverfit that embracing the publicity would mean I could get the Silverfit message – it's never too late to start – out more widely. Talking to the Women's Institute, I realised they were about much more than jam and cakes these days, and that a motivational talk with a few fun photos could spread the Silverfit message further.

I also had the privilege of joining Dr Noel Collins, a psychiatrist specialising in old age, and Mary Jordan who recently wrote a book together on dementia, *The D Word – Rethinking Dementia*. Noel was another Serpentine RC member whom I had met out in Lanzarote. Together Mary and Noel were addressing a conference for carers of patients with dementia and wanted me to promote the message that it's never too late to start exercising to their carers. Hearing their advice to the audience – all of whom were facing such an awful situation when their partners were no longer the same person as they were, and depleted by the responsibilities they were unexpectedly facing – I vowed that Silverfit would work with other specialist groups to play a part in ensuring that such carers also had the space, time and opportunity to stay physically active. It would be essential that Silverfit sessions enabled a flexible approach, for carers to turn up when they could, knowing that their friends would welcome them back. Or even for a carer to be able to come and take part in an activity such as tai chi, whilst their partner sits at the side and happily watches.

It was such a privilege when the Cabinet Office, guiding the consultation and subsequent launch of the Sports Minister's New Sports Strategy, with a new focus on wellbeing, sent cameras out to interview me, and film me doing press-ups under Vauxhall Bridge!

The impact of all the interviews I have done, the magazine features ranging from the *Evening Standard* to *Audi Magazine*, from *At Home with Gloria Hunniford* to a Marathon Talk podcast, breakfast TV or the 'This Girl Can' video are less measurable than the number of people attending a Silverfit event. It is great, though, that the radio and TV stations, magazines and podcasts want to feature good news stories about ageing healthily. I hear so often the word inspirational. I don't feel inspirational but if someone's mum, neighbour or gran is motivated to get out and exercise just a bit more, even walking just that bit faster for a hundred yards or so, and make new friends, countering social isolation at the same time, then I count that as a fantastic result. But I am not sure my grandchildren anticipated the embarrassment of their 'Mad Granny'. I doubt they would have given 'informed consent'.

10

Age is just a number

On 24 March 2013, I hit the magic age of seventy. The brilliant and memorable birthday celebrations were down in the Churchill War Rooms. Friends came from far and wide, to such a great party venue in the famous Plant Room 7. The caterers again provided a selection of dishes from my grandmother's recipe book, and friends and family also brought the odd plate from her chapter on savouries. My daughter-in-law Angela provided some stunning decorations and it was a great night.

For a triathlete, or a runner, a milestone birthday is also celebrated for reaching a new five-year age group, offering new goals and challenges as the potentially youngest members of the group. That year, although I was excited to be in a new age band, I did wonder if we were the only people who look forward to being that year older. To enter a race knowing that you are the youngest and, therefore, hopefully one of the fastest or fittest, is motivating. However, while I can see that in the age brackets below mine, in running as well as cycling and triathlon, there are significantly more women competing, which is great, it seems those of us over seventy are few and far between.

I needed a major event to challenge me. I deliberated long and hard. Given the huge doubts about my knees, including grade-three arthritis and the lack of any ACLs, I had assured the whole world that Kona in 2010 was my last Ironman. I had convinced myself that era in my life was over.

But was it? Or did I want to prove all the research I was gathering for Silverfit – that it is never too late to start, and age is just a number? I reflected on the risks to my knees and the chances of bringing forward the day I would need surgery.

I had gone to support Steve at Ironman Lanzarote four times, and had raced twice myself, in 2009 and 2010. I loved the dramatic island: the volcanic scenery, the architectural influence of César Manrique, the sandy beaches on one side and waves crashing onto volcanic rocks on the other. In October 2012 I had gone back to support two of my RAAM friends doing the Half Ironman, and envied their time on the bike. I had gone up the famous Tabeyeso climb to cheer them on near to the top. I was wearing my red Serpie gear and many came past calling out 'You Serpies, you get every-where!' or, when they recognised me, 'Why aren't you doing it?' My resolve was weakening. Could I build up enough strength in the muscles supporting my knees to enable me to complete the marathon? Crucially, could I improve my swim and bike split to give me sufficient time to walk/run the marathon and so minimise the damage?

The registration list for Ironman Lanzarote 2013 was almost full. It was a challenge, and now was the moment of decision. I signed up, justifying my actions with the fact that I might be able to get some of my money back if I later told them that I had a worsening knee problem. I was navigating advice from all areas: Kate, my daughter-doctor, reminding me that seventy-year-old joints are not made for running marathons, particularly when you already have problems; and Elaine, my physio, reminding me that, at some point, I would need knee surgery. But Steve had the loudest voice, saying, 'Go for it, I'll come out and support.'

Crucially, did I have the time to devote to the training? I now had control of my own diary for self-employed work as a social work consultant – although I was setting up Silverfit too. Life was going to be very full, but with careful planning, I told myself, everything would be fine.

Annie Emmerson had set me a six-month training plan, and Elaine kept reminding me of the importance of building up my glutes and hamstrings to support my knees to minimise the play between the arthritic bones and not to aggravate the arthritis further. But Annie and Elaine are optimists. They both insisted I could do it even though I had to work on my core and balance. Then there was the third discipline – the swimming. Oh dear, the swimming. I needed to do eight miles per week minimum, including endurance and speed work. I have no problems with the long, slow sessions of any discipline. It's the painful speed work I shy away from. Occasionally, Annie would drag me down to the pool for horrendous sessions of 10 × 25m, or even 10 × 50m. Her coach Brett Sutton, she would tell me, used to set her 100 × 25m sessions.

With cheap flights to Faro, I managed a couple of long weekends biking in the slightly warmer climate of the Algarve. There is a great Specialized bike-hire shop, Bike Algarve, five minutes from the airport – they even keep my pedals there for me! I could cycle on the unspoilt terrain, roads with hardly any traffic, hilly routes, long steady climbs and fabulous descents on good-quality, wide roads. There was a great café at the top of the first major climb out of Faro on the N2, the empty, main road to Lisbon (now replaced by the Autoroute), which took you through some fabulous scenery including the cork-oak forests – what an impact there must have been on this local community when screw-top wine bottles came into use, replacing the need for cork, or when all the traffic was diverted to go via the new motorway. In this area, there are remarkably few cyclists, although I have come across the odd national team out training. I wonder why the Algarve is not more popular, compared with the packed roads and hordes of cyclists in Majorca. I have often spent several days there, riding alone but loving it. I am sure I am not riding as fast as I would in a group, but I love it.

Following this, I went on the Serpentine trip to Club La Santa. There were ten days of biking bliss and the odd dip in the 50-metre pool. And then on to Steve Trew and Dan Bullock's camp in Cesenatico. I left a great fun group in Italy a week early, and came home to grab my stuff to head back to Lanzarote for the Ironman.

On arriving in Lanzarote, despite seeing friendly faces and such a familiar race course, big nerves still kick in. Hotel Fariones, the official race hotel, where I was staying, over-looks the seafront so it was on to the beach at 9 a.m. the day before the race, for one last swim in the ocean with my new wetsuit, one with great orange fins on the arms to optimise the catch of water. This will probably become illegal soon. Although it's a mixed blessing for me, after 1900m my arms get so tired I think I lose any advantage as I fail to catch the water.

In the last nerve-racking days, the main high street trans-forms into the race venue. The race is part of the island's economy and reputation, bringing athletes in for training all year, and absolutely everyone is so, so enthusiastic. They are particularly encouraging of an older woman, though most assumed I was there as a supporter. There was a comment at registration when one of the staff from Club La Santa, who knew me from the Serpentine trip, asked if I was over to support. She was totally shocked when I said I was actually doing the Ironman. So much for stereotypes.

Steve arrived: this time, just to support me. We ate together, but had no alcohol for those last few days – well, perhaps just one glass of wine on the penultimate night, which is generally regarded as the important night to get a good long sleep, as sleep is often more disturbed the last night before a race. By now, although I was more familiar with the routine of planning bags, setting out kit, race numbers etc, and ensuring the bike is race-ready, the anxiety level doesn't diminish. Tension is always in the air. It is a big, big day for every single competitor, the fruition of so many hours of blood, sweat and tears. Ironman races may rightly be viewed as 'dumbed down' over the last few years, as more competitors take part at a less elite level, and are not aiming to go under a twelve-hour finish time, but that is not to underestimate the effort that every single person has made, whatever their goal.

Finally, race day dawned. Hotels serve breakfast from 4 a.m. onwards, and arriving in the dining room at five, I realised that I was the last competitor down. It was raining. Lanzarote weather statistics promise only 2mm of rain during the whole of May and this was it. It really was raining hard – probably the whole month's quota fell in an hour at the start of the Ironman. I knew that would cause difficulties on the bike. But I breakfasted in the quiet dining room, having my usual – an egg, some smoked salmon, toast and peanut butter and loads of black coffee. Still almost pitch dark, I went down to my bike to check the tyres. I made sure my High5 Extreme drink was on board, and my energy gels were strapped to the bike, with one ibuprofen and one paracetamol tablet taped on too, in case I was in serious pain partway through – in the heat my wide feet swell and can sometimes get really sore. At 6.30 a.m., with wetsuit on and BodyGlide applied where needed, I was one of the last down onto the beach. Dawn slowly breaking, thousands of black rubber souls were assembled silently under a huge inflatable gantry. Is there time for a quick pop down in the water for a warm-up? I went in very, very briefly, enough to follow Dan Bullock's advice and do a 'flush out' of the water from my wetsuit, pushing it around to get that seal to prevent further water loading, and to tell myself it wasn't really that cold. I thought of a Serpie friend, Chrissie, who completed the Channel swim, and was able to visualise a furnace within her, warming her up.

All the time the noise and tension were building up, with commentary on loudspeakers. I thought I heard a reference to an old woman of seventy here for the first time, and opening up a new age-group category for women. Was that really me, I asked myself, but I kept my head down. There was jostling in the androgynous black-rubbered pack, but my aim was to be at the back, not the front. And finally, the countdown and we were off, shuffling herd-like down the beach. We then ran into the shallow water, and as it got deeper and we could no longer stand up, we all took those first few strokes, inadvertently hitting other swimmers but keeping our heads down, and goggles safe for about twenty metres. And then it calmed and the real swim began, most of the other swimmers already out in front of me. There was no need to sight on the big red buoy three hundred metres straight out to sea; I just followed the pack and stayed close to the line of buoys to my left. Again there was that weird sensation of swimming over a cameraman, his oxygen-tank bubbles rising to the surface.

I know the theory of drafting – swimming on someone's

toes and saving 10 per cent of energy from their displacement of the water – but I have never really mastered that skill. Following closely behind someone doing breaststroke makes some sense, because their direction is perfect, but their kicking can be erratic. But as I reached the deeper water and the colourful fish below, and the row of buoys to hold on to for a very brief rest, I knew why I had come back to Lanzarote again. I was realising, too, that, for the first time, I was not the last swimmer. There were several behind me. Maybe this was all down to the orange fins on my wetsuit, or maybe, just maybe, those training miles had paid off. Finally, at the far extremity of the course, another left turn and I was on the way back, diagonally to the start point, to complete that first lap, sighting on the wonderfully visible view of the Hotel Fariones.

By this time I was being lapped by the race leaders, their accompanying boats taking a route closer to the shore than the swimmers I was following. Did they know something we didn't? Was it the current? Was it a more direct line than the buoys were indicating? I've no idea, but I followed their route on the second lap. If only I could swim half as fast.

At the end of the first lap, I staggered out onto the beach, where a tactful marshal enquired whether I was finishing, or if I had another lap still to do. It's never easy standing up after an hour of horizontal exertion. Whilst all around me people were finishing their swim, yanking wetsuits off and running hell for leather up the beach to get their bikes, I turned and stepped gingerly back into the water for another 1900 metres – another hour. Could I really do it? I was seventy after all. The mind games continued until a I reached the first red buoy again, and made the left turn to begin that long straight kilometre, the shoal of fish below, the support of canoeists and the positive realisation that I was over halfway through an Ironman swim. Counting has always helped me: 10 per cent done and only 90 per cent to go, a hundred and fifty strokes to the next boat, four hundred strokes to the next buoy. Somehow, I turned the final corner and followed the diagonal back to the gantry, sensing the current was helping me home. You know you are almost there when the sand below comes into sharper view, the patterns in the surface fascinatingly elaborate. I had almost finished the swim, and in well under two hours. I was so appreciative of Dan Bullock, Steve Trew and all the others who had helped me with my swimming technique, bearing in mind that ten years earlier I couldn't even do front crawl. The euphoria of finishing the swim is unique. The photo Steve took as I staggered out of the water probably says it all: jubilation.

The worst part was over. I went into the first marquee to change into my bike gear. A volunteer, Debbie, the owner of the Verde Mar restaurant in La Santa village, was standing in the entrance, counting us in. Such is the island commitment to their Ironman. She looked amazed: 'I wasn't expecting you yet; you're ten minutes early. And you're not even the last swimmer out of the water this year.' Now, that really was a compliment. With help, I eased my wetsuit off and then covered myself in sunscreen. I was handed my number and my bike bag, which had everything I needed for the long, long ride. My bike was racked a long way from the beach and I started to walk slowly through the fenced-off transition towards it. I'd finished the swim ahead of schedule and the 2 hours, 20 minutes swim cut-off – there was no hurry!

I passed Kenneth Gasque, who also seemed genuinely relieved to see me out of the swim. He congratulated me, we discussed the swim a bit before he tentatively suggested, 'It is a race, and maybe you should go a bit faster in transition.' I had been content to have a rest and a chat. Despite the tough terrain and the winds, Kenneth is the reason that so many of us go back, year after year, to the warmth and family feel of the Lanzarote Ironman.

So, finally, I was on the bike. What a feeling it was – pedalling rhythmically along the familiar high street, with loads of supporters cheering me on, many recognising me as the old woman from the previous Ironman Lanzarote film, or maybe because I had been there so many times – or, more likely, because they knew I was one of the last to get out on the bike route. I'd hear 'Go Eddie!', or occasionally that inexplicable American salute, 'Way to go!' Sure, I had 220.2 kilometres still to go.

My other personal goal was to get every Lanzarote policeman to smile. Sometimes in other races, without the island pride of Lanzarote, the police look so bored and bad-tempered. So I set out to get every policeman I passed to smile. There were an awful lot of them, at every junction, but they did all smile as I cheerily waved, or shouted out the odd 'Gracias'. Poor guys. I knew it was such a boring job waiting for the slower athletes to pass through. I know that feeling, from marshalling and organising races myself, of the frustrations of having to wait for the last competitor to come home, however much you admire their spirit and determination to finish.

Away from the crowds and the town, the peace kicked in – along with the wind and drizzle. Later that night I learnt that this was one of the windiest Ironman races in its twenty-two-year history. The worst parts were on a couple of the steepest climbs up to Haría and Mirador. There are a few kilometres of main road before that long windy climb up to Yaiza, with the fabulous views looking sideways down to the blue sea and cliffs. The route bypasses Yaiza and past an elevated roundabout where, down below, the other exit leads up to

Fire Mountain. Dozens of the Ironman cyclists were already battling up that hill, but I still faced over an hour of riding as I tried to work out whether they were going directly into the wind. Repeatedly I asked myself why I was doing this, and told myself that the next five hours or so were going to hurt. If I had known it was going to be a further seven hours on the bike I might have had second thoughts.

But then came my answer – that lovely long fast downhill towards Playa Blanca, the exhilaration spoilt only by the sight of so many cyclists struggling back up the hill towards me. Only slowly did it dawn on me that they weren't going so slowly because of the gradient, they were battling into a headwind. And I realised why I was going so fast down the hill. How could I have thought my speed was due to all my training and the euphoria of finishing the swim and being out on the bike?

The El Golfo loop is a high point of the ride, starting off with the beauty of the desalination plant that is so vital for water supply of the island, the fantastic deep blue water, huge waves crashing onto the dramatic black volcanic rock formations and all the surrounding terrain of a lava field in the National Park. And this year, after Ros Young's Vines and Volcanoes talk for Serpentine a couple of months earlier, I was now able to identity different lava, and appreciate the consequences of the 1730–6 volcanic eruptions that led to the lava of this fabulous National Park and that covered of 25 per cent of the island, including eleven villages. As I finished my bottle of High5 and downed another gel in the hope that I'd get a sufficient caffeine boost for Fire Mountain, I grabbed a fresh bottle at the drink station and reflected how lucky I was, and what fun I was having in such a stunningly beautiful location.

As I finished the El Golfo loop and hit the hill, I remembered why I had been bombing so fast downhill, faster than

ever before. Going back up was really tough, the gentle
incline seemed endless. Then finally, a turn-off and I was out
of the headwind and riding up the straight hill towards Fire
Mountain. It was a long, long drag against the nightmare
wind. Again I was counting – I knew the hill so well, I broke
it down into eleven stages. To get to the top of the next plateau,
I wondered if I should stand or if I should save my legs and
pull from the glutes from a seated position. More mind games.

At last, I reached the entrance to Fire Mountain. I cycled
past the lovely coffee shop built into the volcanic rock, and
the long row of camels waiting to offer rides up the mountain.
I promised myself I'd try a sedentary lifestyle one day.

After this it was mostly downhill for many miles, past
Club La Santa at Famara Beach, then it was up and up and up
again. A sight that really motivated me was a car parked in a
layby on a hill with Abba blaring, and a mum and her three
kids dancing to the music, waving cheerleader pompoms and
shouting encouragement to every rider. What a great idea,
and what a difference it made at a crucial point. They were
not just there to cheer their dad on, but were waiting around
for some of the slower oldies. Lovely, and so typical of the
Lanzarote island support.

I knew that final big push up to Haría and Mirador so well,
and yet again there was a headwind. Just after the steepest bit
of the ride, through the countryside, there is a high wall on
the left and suddenly it ends and there is a view I have dreamt
about – it's my phone screen saver – the most fabulous scene
of Graciosa Island in a sea of blue. It is no wonder Manrique
created one of his most notable buildings at Mirador del Rio.
Both the café and the outside balcony are built into the rocks,
with the stunning views of Graciosa Island. We have all biked
past many, many times without realising what a fantastic café
lay below.

And then down, down and round and down again, as fast as I dared, for mile after fantastic mile on a brilliantly re-surfaced, traffic-free road. With none of the potholes of the Surrey Hills to fear or induce caution. I was on the main highway on the leeward side of the island; the wind now was not so bad.

As I finally rolled down the last hill into Puerto del Carmen, I was one of the last, but not the very last. On the beach side of the road dozens of runners in various states of depletion, dehydration and exhaustion were running in the blazing afternoon sun. Such varied paces – not easy for any of them. Many still found a tiny bit of energy to wave at me, or put a thumb up.

I reached the timing mat. What a relief to get off my bike, albeit so, so stiffly. Could I really run, jog or walk a marathon? But the bike was taken from me and racked. And there in the transition area were some of the competitors who had finished the race, medals hanging proudly around their necks, just going into the beer tent. They were the ten-hour finishers and I was about to start a marathon. Envy was an understatement. Could I really do this? Maybe that is the real point of decision in an Ironman, as you wonder just how much energy has been sapped by that relentless afternoon wind.

It was a long, long transition to collect my run bag, put my shoes on and start back out. However, I was finally on the run, number belt to the front, through the phalanx of support and immediately up what feels like a steep, short hill but is probably only a gentle slope. It was cooler now – at least there is one advantage to getting out on the run as the sun goes down. For the first time, I realised how late it was – it was 5 p.m. – and just how long that bike ride had taken. It had been at least an hour longer than I had hoped, putting me under pressure to walk/run the marathon by midnight.

This was the moment of truth. Could these dodgy knees manage a marathon? Had I done enough strengthening exercises? I ran past some of the shops and bars, their main clientele not yet in for their first drink, and then I was into a stretch of road parallel to the airport runway, planes taking off and landing. There were no crowds here. This was the moment, I told myself, to try the walk/run. My watch measured a speed of 8.5kph – not bad, but if I ran it was ten minutes per kilometre.

Suddenly, there was Steve. He'd found a quieter spot to cheer me on. He joined me alongside, for fifty metres or so, though he couldn't keep up with my walking pace. 'Mum, you are actually walking quite fast, but you do need to start running again now – or you won't make tonight's cut-off.' The more distance I covered, the less I was able to calculate. I knew I had to finish by midnight to be an Ironman, but it was all about balancing the damage to the knee versus the time limit. All of my mind games and internal debates were taking place without me realising that so many people were also anxiously watching my times online, especially back at camp in Cesenatico, worrying as my pace slowed that I might not make it. Little did they realise how finely I was timing it, anxiously tracking with Steve when I saw him at various points on the run route whether I could make it before midnight, or if I could walk just a bit more instead of having to run.

As darkness descended, the whole route became more magical, more fun, with sparkling lights and what seemed like the whole island out to support. I could see the swim buoys were still in place as I ran along the beach road. Did I really manage to swim that far? At the turn-around point there was a loud, pavement disco outside a shop – any music with a strong beat is so motivating, so I asked if they would play Queen's 'Don't Stop Me Now' on my way back. The beat and the lyrics of that song have always energised me. They were brilliant: as I returned twenty minutes later, I jogged past waving to the sound of Queen and my speed leapt up.

As you complete each lap you collect a coloured wristband, so you know how many are left – and you always know, from their wristbands, how far ahead others are. One lap to go: brilliant, well done. I was surprised at how many people seemed to know me, or maybe just wanted to offer encouragement to an old woman, still without any wristband. But what camaraderie and support, running or walking. Sometimes, when walking, I would overtake those jogging, less and less energetically. At this point, competitiveness has disappeared – we're all in this together and we are having fun. There was none of the isolation that came with Kona, along the Queen K highway at night, with just a head torch for company.

What a privilege it was to come face to face with Gordon Haller, the very first Ironman winner from 1978, out on the run. He didn't know me, but he recognised a fellow oldie – even though he is seven years younger. At the awards ceremony the following day it was lovely to hear Gordon describe Ironman Lanzarote as the best he had ever done. It really is a compliment, says something about the island's support, the warmth, the organisation and all of the competitors.

Gordon and I crossed paths for the last time right out at the far end of the run loop. I was probably twenty minutes ahead, and we were both walking as we high-fived each other. Finally, it was back to the noise and the loudspeakers revving up as I came down the last slope, with all the supporters still out at nearly midnight. At last, under the gantry and there was Kenneth, waiting with my friend Isabelle to congratulate me, and give me my medal. The oldest woman to have done Ironman Lanzarote, though I realised my time of 16 hours, 43 minutes – just seventeen minutes to the midnight deadline – was cutting it a bit fine.

The celebratory supper and awards ceremony the next day was emotional, a celebration of my age. As I stood on that podium, trophy held high, everyone standing to cheer this old woman, I realised the power of the message they were all sending me about healthy ageing. Could I use this knowledge, and enthusiasm for Silverfit, to make that crucial difference for our ageing population, using exercise to have fun and make new friends to share the fun? Did I have the skills to reach out and optimise the message that it is never too late to start, even, with advice from a GP, when we are already suffering from injuries or chronic disease?

11

Blood is thicker than water

With the combination of setting up Silverfit, my own training and helping to organise the Serpentine trip to Lanzarote, not to mention having a social life, my life was pretty full and I questioned whether I was giving enough time to my children and grandchildren and their ups and downs. Did I have too much on my plate to do justice to any part? How did my grandchildren really view their mad gran and her crazy lifestyle? Not untypically, I failed to resolve the pressures, knowing that my own level of physical activity and the fun I was having in life was itself providing an example to Silverfitters, and even the family, that seventy was just a number.

While 2013 had the potential to be an insanely busy year with some great opportunities to share with the family, I never dreamt it would be so exciting, or so much fun. The ITU World Triathlon Championships were due to be held in Hyde Park – my nearest and favourite park, and the home to both Serpentine Running Club and Serpentine Swimming Club. It seemed a shame not to be able to participate, so I resolved I would try to qualify. Although I had raced for Great Britain at the World Duathlon Championships, I had rarely competed over the Olympic triathlon distance (1.5k swim, 40k bike, 10k run). I certainly hadn't qualified to represent the GB age-group team. I would have to go up to Chester for the Deva Triathlon, which was the designated qualifying race, at the beginning of June.

A minor problem was that only a week earlier I would hopefully have completed Ironman Lanzarote. I could hear people saying that seventy-year-old bodies were not really meant for this and that the minimum recovery time should be four weeks. But when I signed up for the Deva Triathlon, it looked as though I might be the only one in the 70–75 age group. To qualify for the World Championships age-group team you have to do a race over the same distance, and come in the top four or five of your age group. So, 'You've only got to finish,' I told myself, 'and you'll get to race in Hyde Park, and then you can relax and watch the professionals race, including those incredible Brownlee brothers. After all,' I kept repeating to myself, 'it is only Olympic distance, only a 10k run and you will have a whole week for rest and recovery after the Ironman.'

But there was another problem: the swim in the River Dee. At the beginning of June the water flowing through Chester would be cold. I realised that meant I had to get in some practice in colder water. In other words, I knew I had to be brave and go for those early-morning swims, 6.30 to 9.30 a.m. in the Serpentine.

Deva Triathlon proved to be a lovely race, with a great atmosphere and a fabulous run route through Grosvenor Park. The River Dee starts in Snowdonia and flows eastwards. The current going out felt strong, and for the last four hundred metres before the turnaround I despaired, knowing

I was making very slow progress. Maybe all those pessimistic people were right, and I was too tired. Perhaps older bodies really do need several·weeks to recover. For this final stretch, there were only a few people left swimming in my direction and most of the swimmers had turned around and were on their way back, on the other side of the river. But as I finally reached the large turn buoy I too experienced the compensation of a speedy return back to base, the current now strongly in my favour. I finished the swim, was on my bike and then on to the undulating run. I completed Deva Triathlon, the one and only competitor in my age group, and so it was on to the World Championships in August.

Not long after the Deva Triathlon came an email, out of the blue, from the BBC producer Sarah Richardson. She was going to be covering the two-day event in Hyde Park. We age-groupers would be going off early on the Sunday morning, finishing just ahead of the start of the male professional athletes' race, where the real world champions, including the Brownlee brothers, would be competing. Sarah told me she had read the *Guardian* article, and seen I had qualified at Deva, so wanted to film some of my preparation. With less than a week to go, we arranged to meet for a photoshoot at Hampton Pool, a fantastic open-air heated pool and the scene of one of my first triathlons.

I knew Annie was going to be doing the live commentary of the race so I thought it would be fun if she could join us for the shoot. It proved to be such an enjoyable day. All action and lots of fun. A cameraman and a producer filmed my far-from-perfect swimming in the lido, insisting that my hand with the Union Jack painted on my nails was visible, and Annie was advising me from the side of the pool. Then we all went over to Bushy Park to film a bit of running. Several deer were watching on, motionless and clearly nonplussed by the repeat takes as Annie and I jogged up and down past them, again, again and yet again. Then we went to Herne Hill velodrome, a venue at the 1948 Olympics and training ground for so many of our top cyclists, including Bradley Wiggins. I often joined Crystal Palace Triathletes for their weekly evening road bike sessions, so knew the place well. The whole day of filming was so enjoyable, and I thought that perhaps with this film I could make a tiny difference by motivating a few oldies who wanted to get a bit more active after seeing the fun I was having. I hadn't reckoned on two million viewers.

The race in Hyde Park lived up to my dreams. I wasn't worried about winning my age group, just thrilled to be taking part. Still, I was probably taking everything too casually and was late leaving home and cycling for fifteen minutes up to registration. Punctuality has never been my forte, and I was horrified to reach the transition area and find it closed. All those other competitors had come from all over the world and had their bikes safely racked, but I hadn't been able to get there in time. Seriously embarrassed, I wondered if this was the moment to play the 'confused oldie' card, having lost my way in Hyde Park. Fortunately, I found a marshal who let me in to rack quickly, sort my stuff out and grab my wetsuit. That was all too close for comfort.

The ground felt really cold as we made the long trek from transition down to the swim start but I wasn't expecting the great news that the swim distance had been shortened to 750 metres because of the combined low water and air temperature. Now that was a real result: only half the distance, in a lake I knew well. I loved every minute of the swim, and with roads closed to traffic as we biked out to Park Lane, I was having a ball, cheered on by so many Serpentine members marshalling around the course. I did wonder and worry about how much it must cost to close such crucial roads in the centre of London, with all those smiling police, and how many people had been affected by the inevitable traffic jams. But for me, it was unbelievable – down to Green Park, around Buckingham Palace and the Victoria Memorial, then back underneath Wellington Arch at the centre of Hyde Park Corner. We sped along the closed park roads, up over the bridge across the Serpentine to a turnaround and then back, past the finish arch and out for another two unbelievable laps. Time was irrelevant. I was on such a high, and it was a fantastic, memorable experience for all of us. As a local, surrounded by family and club members, it was a humbling and incredible privilege. Then finally on to the last lap of the run, a slight diversion and it was down the finishing straight, hearing the familiar tones of Steve Trew doing the live commentary. Yet again he lost no opportunity to tell the world how old I was.

There too, to my surprise, was the BBC TV crew recording me as I came through the finish gantry. I had had no idea when the film was actually going out, so I was astonished to learn that the whole film was actually broadcast very shortly after I finished and just ahead of the main race – they really didn't have long to edit and add that bit to the filming they had done earlier in the week. It was watched by a huge audience that had tuned in to watch the Brownlees' race. It was great, too, that the film and then the professionals' race was introduced by Chrissie Wellington, the multiple Ironman World Champion whom I had known for years, saying I had inspired her! What a great and diverse community the triathlon family is, and we are still in touch, exploring ways of encouraging older people to have a go at Parkruns.

Reading the responses to the *Guardian* blog and seeing the reactions to the film, I was beginning to realise that the voices of older, fitter people might have a greater impact on the sedentary, ageing population than younger Lycra-clad, slim people in gyms. As a charity, Silverfit was starting to feel its way, holding weekly sessions in Hyde Park and Burgess Park, changing the lifestyles of oldies and facilitating socialising, enabling them to have the fun I have had.

Steve had been part of my Ironman history, but what a fun experience it was, a year later, to be offered the opportunity to compete in the New York City Triathlon in a team of eight with both of my sons, and a couple of their friends, my son-in-law and my adopted son Chris. Both Steve and Gary were confident they would beat their seventy-one-year-old mother, although I consoled myself by reflecting that their superiority was all down to the hours I had spent encouraging them as children to feel more water-confident. As I flew to New York, the fear of jumping into the Hudson River kept creeping into my thoughts. Could I do it? What else was also in that water? How high was that jump? How would I ensure my goggles stayed on when I jumped in?

I guess it was the fear of that big jump that made me walk alone, west from our hotel in Second Avenue and across Manhattan, a couple of days before the race to view the swim start. As I strolled across Fifth Avenue and then on to Times Square, memories flooded back, along with a few tears, of the family holiday we had taken in New York many years ago, when Phil had suggested that rather than get a boat trip around Manhattan, we would all walk from the tip of the island all the way up to the top of Central Park. With anxiety building up, I arrived at the vast Hudson River, stretching out and across into the distance. Could I really swim in that huge river? I decided I had to see the pontoon – the start barge, as they call it – from which I knew I would have to jump. I turned northwards and walked up along the pavement parallel to the Hudson. It is an incredibly busy river with large and small boats criss-crossing each other. Could I really swim down the middle?

One of my first sights was the USS *Intrepid*, a huge former aircraft carrier from the Second World War and now an air, sea and space museum, moored next to the bank. My only thought was that if this huge boat came up the Hudson, the river must be so, so deep. On I walked, with ever-increasing trepidation and panic. I kept reminding myself of Dan Bullock's advice for open-water swimming: 'Overcoming your fears comes from the confidence of knowing you have done it in training or replicated conditions in a less stressful environment.' That advice wasn't going to help me now as I couldn't put it into practice.

The feeling of being in a washing machine, with bodies swimming over and under me, thrashing arms everywhere, at the beginning of a race isn't ever a problem for me as I always lurk around at the back. But that Saturday I would be jumping in with nine others, to be followed only twenty seconds later by another ten swimmers. I hadn't practised that. Nor had I ever swum in the Hudson, or seen the course. By Dan's criteria I had done nothing to overcome my fears. The pictures on the website show people diving in. That would have been a complete no-no for me. I can't dive. Fortunately, only the professionals are permitted to dive in; all the rest have to jump.

Finally, as I walked further northwards, I saw a large newly erected board at the junction with 81st Street that read SWIM FINISH. And as I reached it, I gasped aloud with relief. I could suddenly see a row of tiny buoys stretching ahead of me in a long line – a line a mile long. It was such a welcome sight. Connected by rope, those buoys were marking off a swim lane in the Hudson. It was only about ten metres wide and was adjacent to the bank below me. All those huge boats ploughing up and down were on the far side of the buoys.

My fears almost evaporated. Now I could see that the

swim was just a mile of liquid tranquillity parallel to the
bank. On race day there would surely be loads of canoeists
on the other side of the lane, protecting the swimmers from
any passing boats. Maybe, too, it wouldn't be as deep at the
side of the river. As I peered down over the wall, I could see
black rocks below – I relaxed, realising that I could always
climb onto them and wait to be rescued. So just two fears
remained: the jump, and the contamination of the water. As
every astonished New York cab driver had commented to me,
as a English oldie, 'Gee, have you come all this way across the
big pond to swim in the Hudson with all those dead bodies,
rats, and dumped chemicals?'

Anxiously, I paced out the mile upriver, past the endless
transition area that had already been set up in readiness for the
bikes. Finally, there it was: the start barge. It was an empty
pontoon, two metres wide and sticking out at right angles for
about ten metres. This was the jump, and it was only a metre
or so above water level. I could do that. Yes I could. I walked
back to the hotel feeling considerably relieved, stopping at
St Patrick's Cathedral for a brief Mass. It happened to be in
Polish for a sector of the local population, but the order was
exactly the same as Mass at home. Then, memorably, my first
sight of the new Freedom Tower, where the Twin Towers
had been. I had been to New York quite a few times before,
and had social work friends living nearby. I had known one
of the local Northamptonshire badminton lads, Geoff, who
had died there, and I had gone to the Requiem Mass for
him, with no body. I reflected on how his family could have
coped with that level of trauma and loss. Somehow my own
loss seemed easier to make sense of. I walked on, and back to
join our family triathlon group, to relax, and have the odd
drink to reduce the panic.

*

All triathlons are complicated, and for the New York triathlon there were different start points for the swim, the bike and the run, with lengthy transitions to be negotiated. No one in the family rates my logistical skills. Organising the wetsuit, goggles and hat at the swim start, the bike shoes, sunglasses, helmet and race number in the bike racking area, and ensuring a pair of running shoes were available in the right place, not to mention a numbered bag containing warm, dry clothing that would be transported from the swim start to the finish line in Central Park, was an organisational challenge.

I had sourced great turquoise T-shirts and vests for the team, and had arranged to have the name of our chosen charity, Action Duchenne, printed on them. It was an unusual, bright colour, so we were absolutely astounded to see that all seven hundred New York City Triathlon volunteers had shirts of exactly the same colour. How could I have predicted that?

Unusually, the race briefing was compulsory and held on the hour, every hour, with your hand stamped as you emerged. Wisely but unusually, you weren't allowed to register or collect bags for the race unless you could prove you had been to the briefing. Then came the body-marking. Your age was written in waterproof pen on your left calf. Comments by the marking volunteer on my fat, or muscular calf muscles, as they flatteringly called them, led me to quip, 'Just you wait till you see my two sons' calf muscles.'

Then we had to rack our bikes by 5 p.m. on the Saturday. That was a memorable, scary cycle ride for the six of us, across the route I had walked the day before. Manhattan traffic is dramatically different from traffic in London. There was not a bike to be seen between the aggressive cars, and no cycle lanes, just endless traffic lights – we were weaving our way through the un-cycle aware and un-cycle friendly traffic on a Saturday afternoon in downtown New York.

Sunday was race day. As I was in one of the earlier waves I was up at 4 a.m., carb-loading, and then into a packed coach to take us over to transition. It was eerily quiet. I checked everything was in place before starting the unusual mile-plus walk to the swim start, barefoot along the pavement, carrying bag no. 2 and my wetsuit, goggles and the white swimming hat that denoted I was in the over-fifties women's wave.

Close to the swim start was an impressive array of loos – a facility all too often in short supply. With wetsuits on, we were ushered into pens stretching right down alongside the river, grouped according to colour of hat and age. All the women were together. I marvelled at the efficiency of the water entry as the race began and the faster guys were off. Ten people at a time were lined up along the pontoon, the timing mat miraculously stretching along the length of the pontoon to record start times and link with the timing chips on our ankles. As the klaxon sounded, ten bodies jumped into the water and started to swim south. They seemed to be swimming fast; I knew they were the faster younger guys. Ten more were already lined up behind them, and twenty seconds later, in they jumped.

My nerves somehow evaporated as my wave moved up in the long queue, until suddenly we were down the ramp and on to the pontoon. A mere forty seconds later I was in place on the start barge, ten seconds to get really, really scared, and then I was off. I was the last of the group to hit the water. It was raining and misty, but I could just see the end point. Anyway, it was a straight line. I sighted on a red light in the distance that seemed to be on the right line, and that kept me close to the line of buoys. I was never a good swimmer, but this was really fun. After only a few minutes the faster swimmers from the next wave – identifiable by their hat colour – were sailing past me. I vaguely noticed that I was keeping up with, and even overtaking, some of the swimmers to my left, nearer the bank, but I knew that the New York City Triathlon encourages novices. Maybe I wouldn't be the last white hat out of the water.

As we swam south, there were loads of canoeists to our right and huge banners on the bank to the left denoting 300m, 600m, 900m, 1200m, and gosh, I was almost there. At the end I scrambled out on a sort of ramp with a handrail and there were three charming, strong guys pulling me out – they must have seen me coming and known I would really need their help!

Then there was the interminable run back to transition, barefoot across gritty tarmac. It felt as though it was at least eight hundred metres as my bike was racked at the far, far end of the transition compound. A quick look at my watch – 19 minutes, 38 seconds for the swim. How could that be possible? I was absolutely certain I couldn't have pressed the start button at the right time – it normally takes me forty-two to forty-five minutes for 1500m. That just could not be right, even if the current was helping me. But never mind, I would get out on the bike, the bit I love, with the feel-good factor of having finished the swim.

Although the course was hillier that I had anticipated, it was a fantastic 40k. I loved every single minute, surrounded by such companionable and courteous women. NYC Tri is proud of its reputation as an accessible race: there were bikes with baskets, mountain bikes, old and young riders, with many racing for charity. I was not, as is usually the case, the slowest bike rider. Indeed, I was actually overtaking many women. As they saw my age marked on my left leg, many women seemed galvanised into action and would overtake me a few minutes later. Most would call out, shouting encouragement: 'Way to go!', 'You've got it!' or 'Good on you, hope I can do it at your age.' The Americans really are so much more outgoing, enthusiastic and vocal in their support. Supporters at the roadside were also shouting encouragement all the way along: 'Good job, good job!' 'Wow, isn't this absolutely fantastic?' I shouted to fellow cyclists as we went over the long traffic-free Henry Hudson Bridge and into the Bronx. This was a high to beat all highs!

And then, I could see the lads coming back towards me on the other side of the road, finding time to wave and shout enthusiastic encouragement. A few miles later, at Gunhill Road in the Bronx, there was a U-turn and I too was cycling back towards downtown New York. Back across the Henry Hudson Bridge and shortly afterwards the skyline of Manhattan came into sight and looked incredible. What a fantastic experience. Finally, I was back in transition, and that long walk through to the very end of the rows of bike racks. Never, ever before had mine been the first bike back onto a rail of ten bikes in transition. Usually, I come back to full rails of bikes – their owners already out on the run.

The first mile was hard, along the crowded 72nd Street to Central Park. Despite the cheering crowds and volunteers, it hurt. My legs were like jelly. 'It's OK,' I told myself, 'you are here for the experience. Accept you have problematic knees and just relax and enjoy.' This was another of the mind games I use when feeling tired or needing an excuse not to push myself. Only when we hit Central Park and I looked quickly back did I realise we had been climbing steadily for the first mile. I relaxed and loved every minute of the run: dozens of volunteers, all so enthusiastically making eye contact with every runner, shouting encouragement. I often heard 'Go Eddie', and would turn to smile appreciatively, before realising there are an awful lot of Eddies in New York, and no one would actually know my name. Could anyone, I wondered, resist a smile at one placard held aloft, reading SMILE IF YOU PEE'ED IN THE HUDSON. As the most efficient way of heating the body inside the wetsuit in the cold water of the Hudson, my guess was that most of us had, adding further to the contamination.

I collected a slip of paper with my efficiently processed split times. Incredibly, I realised for the first time that I really had swum a mile in 17.38. Without realising it, I had clearly optimised the benefit of the current by sticking to the buoy line. Overall I was the first of two in my 70–74 age category – or, as my sons put it, second last! I am now the proud owner of a big red apple trophy. The post-event celebrations were memorable as we explored the nightlife of New York, medals proudly round our necks. A wonderful experience, and I was a very proud mum, especially having beaten one son on the swim! It was fun, too, to go together to get matching tattoos, on a triathlon theme. We compared the pain level in different parts of the body. Mine, just above my right ankle, below my Ironman tattoo, seemed one of the least painful locations.

The following weekend was Prudential RideLondon, a hundred miles on the Olympic route through the Surrey Hills. I was thrilled to be riding it with Gary and my daughter. What a privileged mother. Kate hadn't had any time to train and had never cycled more than twenty-five miles in one go. We all went together, parked a car close to the Emirates Air Line at Greenwich, and had the wonderful experience of crossing the Thames to the Royal Docks, marvelling at the views of the City and the Olympic Park, with our three bikes alongside us in the cable car, and then only a short ride to our different start points in the Olympic Park.

The weather forecast was grim: so grim that the distance was reduced from a hundred miles to eighty-six, missing out two of the major hills, or more importantly, two of the descents. With the high numbers of cyclists, descending on wet, muddy roads would have been lethal.

I have never, ever cycled in weather like it – storms, pouring rain, roads flooded so you couldn't see the pot-holes beneath and accidents that stopped us all for ages in Richmond Park. As an inexperienced cyclist I don't know how Kate survived. All around us was evidence of punctures, punctures and yet more punctures. I have never seen so many upturned bikes at the side of the road. We were very lucky to avoid a flat. The photo of Kate and me riding up the Mall together to the finish remains one of my all-time favourites; Gary, of course, had finished ages earlier.

Sport has given us all a closer link, and triathlon now even extends to two of my grandkids. There was a brief window when my grandson Ben was the right size to have my bike, before he began to tower above me and outgrew my cast-offs. Briefly, too, Tilly was the same shoe size. I had bought a new, expensive pair of running shoes in the right size and right brand, but found they were far too narrow. Fortunately, they fitted Tilly. And now, too, she is on that old bike.

Having set me up as Mad Granny71 on Instagram, Ben then persuaded a few of his friends to like me because, 'poor thing, she hasn't got many friends'. He has waited patiently for me, his Irongran, to cross the finish line of the Christmas Day Parkrun at Bushy Park in double his time – after he completed the 5k in just over seventeen minutes.

It must be so embarrassing for all my grandchildren. When I asked the youngest one, aged twelve, to comment on their mad granny, she said, 'She's crazy.' Asked what made me crazy, she responded, 'You do something that a thirty-year-old would do.' Asked why that was crazy she was clear: 'Cos you are so old.' I was recording her views in a nail bar, with Kate next to her, her beautiful long blue nails drying in front of her. I asked what was embarrassing about me and she said, 'This recording here in the nail bar.' Asked about the experience of spending a day out with her grandmother in London, she said there were a lot of trains and too much walking and it wasn't really a leisurely day at all. Strangely, though, I asked her if she would prefer to have a grandmother sitting in a chair, knitting all day, and I got a firm 'No!' We talked a little about our respective triathlon skills and she claimed that she could run and swim faster than me, but she hesitated longer over the cycling, and finally conceded that I might just be a bit faster.

As with the New York triathlon, there is a sense of privilege of sharing such fun with the family. Our fun, or maybe competitiveness, extends to our Fitbit groups as we struggle to come first, to be the one who's done the most steps at the end of a weekend or a five-day period. I would put my Fitbit around my ankle when on a turbo and be called a cheat. I have not yet found a way to gain steps when I swim – to swim three thousand metres and record fewer than a thousand steps is so frustrating. But overall that competition, when walking gains the optimum steps, is such a healthy incentive to be more active, and be Silverfit.

The key to a healthy older population is making physical activity fun, and finding ways of identifying friends to share the fun. Whilst offering excellent facilities, gyms are still failing to explore the social opportunities which, all our Silverfit data analysis suggests, is the key to retaining that more active lifestyle. We all love a free cup of tea or coffee and a biscuit – maybe a potential offer to increase physical activity? But first I needed to explore the research underpinning healthier ageing.

12

Your health is your most valuable asset

I am part of an ageing population. Twenty millions of us are now aged over fifty – that's more than a third of the UK population – and we are living longer. Although reaching fifty can present challenges in work and home life, facing retirement, menopause, changed lifestyles, living alone, perhaps lacking direction and control, there are also more exciting opportunities than ever before to enjoy life.

I don't just want to live longer. I want to stay fit, healthy and independent, enjoying a good quality of life. I want to minimise the length of time that I'll be relying on others because I am ill, less mobile or depressed. 'Compressed morbidity' is apparently the jargon. I want to slide or swing into my coffin saying 'It's been great!'

As Silverfit was beginning to grow and gain attention, I felt it was important to pull together the research and evidence that show just how much of a killer inactivity can be. Moreover, I wanted to highlight the massive wellbeing benefits of socialising and having fun, plus physical activity and exercise, for the older generation.

With a background in economics, psychology and statistics, I had always been interested in research and its evidence base. My MA at Leicester University had developed to be a PhD when I began to appreciate the significance of the data I had available on the young people who had been placed for adoption, their birth families and their adoptive families. It had taken longer than initially anticipated after Phil's death, but that in a way contributed to the depth of research I could undertake over what was nearly a ten-year period. In my thesis, titled 'JUST Letterbox?', I explored the impact of the new form of indirect contact ('letterbox contact') with birth families, where the local authority managed a system of contact between birth and adoptive families. This sort of 'longitudinal' study is less common, and can be very expensive. Cynically, I knew that behind the headlines lay a variety of influences that could colour the outcomes of research findings: whether it was the size or nature of the sample, the group being used for the study, the funding source or, vitally, the number of variables that might have been present. How, I would ask, did the researchers account for other variables that may have influenced the outcome of specific tests?

My first interest in the research around physical activity came from Professor Harry Burns, then the Chief Medical Officer for Scotland. I had met him at the Parents for Children conference that I was chairing in Edinburgh, on the impact of alcohol on the unborn baby; I had invited him as a guest speaker. He had come into the room prior to the beginning of the conference and, unbeknownst to me, had overheard my earlier conversation with a conference attendee, in which I had been describing my excitement that morning at having got up early to go for a run up to Edinburgh Castle. I had stopped at the top, as a breathtaking dawn was breaking. My only companions, keeping a watchful eye on me, were two urban foxes. Professor Burns gave an illuminating lecture, and as I was seeing him out of the conference room he told me not to give up running and suggested I listen to the Fitness Rocks podcasts. He had, he told me, been a keen runner himself. That was the start of many, many long runs with my iPod. Each week's podcast would have a specific focus and interview on a different research project relating to fitness, with Dr Monte Ladner critically appraising the methodology and strengths or limitations of the research.

I really started to pull the research together after being invited to attend a public health conference in London, on physical activity and the older population. I sought the advice of members of the London South Bank University Sport Science Department, and have valued their support through-out, guiding our data collection and analysis. At that public health conference I head, for the first time, internationally acclaimed speakers and leading researchers – from Dr Mark Hamer describing the lessons being learned from the English Longitudinal Study of Ageing (ELSA)[1] to Dr William Bird of Intelligent Health, Professor Muir Gray and Dr Steven Blair, who caused a storm with his misinterpreted 'fitness matters more than weight' statements.

Why had that huge bank of data about the need to get the older population more physically active not surfaced before? Why were we not hearing about 'the miracle cure of exercise'? Why had my GP not asked me about my level of activity as part of my seventy-year-old health check? I really wanted to play my part as an active oldie in supporting this vital and core message. Accepting that we are living longer means we should live those extra years independently and actively – to enjoy life and have fun, rather than living in discomfort and pain. In other words, being Silverfit.

Life expectancy is increasing. By 2010, the median age at

death had risen to eighty-two for a man and eighty-five for a woman. After accounting for other factors that can affect life expectancy, such as socio-economic status, researchers found that life expectancy was 3.4 years longer for people who reported they achieved the recommended 150 minutes of physical activity per week.[2] People who reported leisure-time physical activity at twice the recommended level gained 4.2 years of life. In general, more physical activity corresponded to longer life expectancy. Although we are living longer, we are spending our later years with more health problems compared with twenty years ago. The massive increase in obesity and type 2 diabetes is having dire and costly consequences. The dilemmas associated with the ageing population raise massive political and economic issues – the choice is between aiming for a frail, disabled and very costly elderly population, and maintaining an active, less isolated, healthy ageing population who only experience real morbidity before death.

Dr Mark Hamer led the team working on the ELSA project. Initiated in 2002, it is one of the first ongoing UK projects to look at the effects of taking up activity later in life. A group of 3400 disease-free participants with an average age of sixty-three were assessed and then studied over eight years to see who aged most healthily without developing major chronic disease, depressive symptoms or physical or cognitive impairment. After adjusting for a number of factors that can have an impact on health (such as age, sex, smoking, alcohol, marital status and wealth), those who became active or continued to be active had significantly improved overall health. This was even true for those who became active relatively late in life.

More and more evidence is coming to light showing that regular physical activity has important and wide-ranging health benefits, as well as reducing the risk of a wide range of chronic diseases. It lowers risk of heart disease and stroke by 35 per cent, type 2 diabetes by 50 per cent, osteoarthritis by 85 per cent, depression by 30 per cent. It is also said to delay dementia by 30 per cent. In 2010, these types of diseases, along with musculoskeletal disorders (mainly lower back pain and falls) were found to be responsible for more than half of all 'years lived with disability'.

Physical inactivity is therefore clearly linked to increased medical costs, and these become ever more significant with increasing age.[3] NHS London estimates that physical inactivity of the over-fifties costs the NHS in London £105 million a year. The costs of type 2 diabetes and resulting complications account for 10 per cent of the total NHS budget – a staggering £14 billion per annum. This takes into account in-patient care, drugs for diabetes and resultant complications, £8.4 billion on absenteeism, and the costs of early retirement, with a commensurate increase in social benefits. Falls, too, have a massive consequence – with further falls ensuing and independence threatened. Those consequences could be dramatically reduced if older people were more active and undertook some minimal strength training.

The evidence builds for an unfit sedentary older population to change their lifestyles and avoid dependence and illnesses. But there are challenges from the economic implications of this. At some point, the cost of pensions for the higher numbers of older people will exceed the benefits or savings to society and the NHS. Can we afford older people? As an economist at heart, I think there are a number of factors that need to be taken into account.

Firstly, we need to consider the tipping point at which the costs of morbidity change. Will health costs increase (because people take longer to die) or stay the same (because they take the same length of time to die, but do it later). Secondly, there is the issue of the extent to which people save for their own retirement. If people expect to live longer, they might make more provision for this. Society also has an attitude towards inheritance that may need to change, to encourage Baby Boomers to spend their savings on their own retirement. Finally, the higher cost of the last weeks of life (intensive care units, hospital stays, hospice care and life-sustaining procedures) could be significantly reduced if patients are able to have effective end-of-life conversations with their doctors.[4]

So all the research indicates that older people must eat more healthily, stop smoking, keep alcohol levels down and, most importantly, stay active. And yet the focus is still not on this final area of prevention. Of course, racing marathons or training for Ironman events is not for everyone. But what is recommended is that over a week your activity should add up to at least 150 minutes of moderate-intensity activity in bouts of ten minutes or more. The accepted way of achieving this is doing about thirty minutes on at least five days a week. Moderate intensity will be something where you feel your heart rate rise. It can be a brisk walk, housework or something more technical. Whatever our age, we should be aiming to minimise the amount of time we spend being sedentary, at the computer as well as in front of the TV. I've set my Garmin watch so that every hour it now vibrates and tells me to MOVE!

I so often hear people say, 'It's too late now to change my lifestyle!' Well, good news resulted from the study of a large cohort of 1861 'very old' men and women born in 1920 and 1921.[5] They were monitored from the age of around seventy years and followed up, exploring the statistics and causes of death and the effect of exercise in people through to age seventy-five and then up to eighty-eight years. It was found that even in this older population regular exercise had an impact on longevity and how well they functioned. People who were physically active at seventy were more likely to be functioning independently. Even those who had begun with more sedentary lifestyles, but later became physically active, had the benefits of living longer. They were measured again at seventy-eight years and those who had remained sedentary were found to have a significantly higher risk of dying and, crucially, were at higher risk of losing the ability to function independently or being disabled by disease. Measured again ten years later, those who were physically active had again benefited: these eighty-eight-year-olds were living longer, and the physical activity had reduced the risk of their frailty. They had higher muscle mass and lower excess body fat. However, the report cautioned that those who stopped exercising reverted to the same level of risk as those who didn't exercise. So use it or lose it!

The key is that once you have started, keep on exercising, even if you feel you can do no more than walking. Dr Hirofumi Tanaka, an expert on ageing athletes, tells us that 'a great deal of the physical effects that we once thought were caused by ageing are actually the result of inactivity'.[6] I love her studies on rats and mice, where more of the variables can be controlled than studies in humans. In one of Dr Tanaka's studies, when elderly rats were given access to running wheels, their leg muscles began sprouting new, hardy populations of satellite cells, those cells that envelop the bodies of their nerve cells, suggesting that their muscles were now able to build and repair themselves effectively.

For all of us, walking is a safe, accessible and low-cost activity and it is known to have great potential to increase physical activity levels in sedentary individuals. Walking speed has been shown to predict 'survival'. For example, an Australian study of 1705 men aged seventy-plus found the mean walking speed was just over 2 miles per hour, or 0.82 metres per second. But survival analysis showed that the men who walked faster than 2 miles per hour were 1.23 times less likely to die than those who walked slower. When their walking speed was 3 miles per hour or greater, none of the men had died. The researchers, with a great sense of humour, concluded that 'the Grim Reaper's preferred walking speed is 0.82 m/s (2 miles (about 3km) per hour) under working conditions. As none of the men in the study with walking speeds of 1.36 m/s (3 miles (about 5km) per hour) or greater had contact with Death, this seems to be the Grim Reaper's most likely maximum speed; for those wishing to avoid their allotted fate, this would be the advised walking speed.'[7]

Now that so many older people have smart phones and wearable technology and apps, we need to persuade every local authority to invest in sensors or a measured Silverfit mile in all their parks and open spaces, in the same way as Intelligent Health, founded by Dr William Bird, are doing with their Beat the Street programme, using activity trackers – 'Beat Boxes' – with sensors on lampposts and bringing together key partners, or promoting competitions within communities or schools, or even care home residents to walk those measured miles, and have fun in the local community.[8]

While the importance of aerobic exercise is clear, there is less emphasis on the strength and balance training recommendations that are also included in the UK Chief Medical Officer's guidelines. Ageing leads to a loss of muscle mass (sarcopenia), and this becomes replaced by fat. Sarcopenia can lead to a loss of independence or significant frailty and these can limit lifestyle. Many studies have reviewed resistance training and they all agree that regular resistance exercise is a potent and effective countermeasure for muscle ageing. It also builds bone. In one study, cohorts of older and younger adults were measured before and after strength training. Initially, the older adults were 59 per cent weaker than the younger, but after six months of training older adults their strength improved significantly, such that they were only 38 per cent lower than the younger adults.[9]

Older adults should aim to do some simple balance and strength training at least twice a week. Just a few exercises to work all the major muscles: hips, legs, back, chest, abdomen, shoulders and arms. Gardening can count, or simply lifting of a couple of cans of baked beans, and a few press-ups and squats.

Alongside the need for strength training is also a need to work on balance. Balance profoundly affects our ability to be mobile and functionally independent, and the term encompasses several different types of control mechanisms for stability: our inner ears, visual information, the proprioceptive system and muscle control. Our brains use information from muscle receptors. With the loss of muscle strength in ageing, balance is reduced. The cerebellum is involved in both maintaining balance and controlling higher mental functions. As that part of the brain declines with age, the detrimental effects on a person's sense of balance become a good measure of future mental decline.

The changes that come with ageing can therefore affect our balance, which in turn affects our likelihood of falling over. In an ageing population, falls for older people represent the greatest cost to the health and care services and are arguably the greatest influence on the quality of life of an individual. Falls attract far less media attention than the risk of cancer or diabetes, and yet falls are the leading cause of both fatal and non-fatal injuries for people over the age of sixty-five. A third of people over sixty-five fall each year, representing half of the hospital admissions for accidental injuries, particularly hip fractures.[10] Half of those with hip fractures never return to their former level of functioning and one in five die within three months as a result of inactivity and factors such as blood clots. Sadly, once older people fall over they become more cautious and the fear restricts their physical activity, muscles are further weakened and the risk of falling increases.

Exercise in general promotes strength, flexibility and balance, and research evidence confirms that pilates and tai chi can also meet the needs for improved balance. In one study, tai chi was associated with a 20 per cent lower risk of falling at least once and a 31 per cent drop in the number of falls.[11]

When we were considering setting up Silverfit, we first thought of the obvious target age as the over-fifties, recognising that the average age of menopause is fifty-one. But in Southwark we were encouraged by Public Health England to include those from the age of forty-five, before women hit the menopause, to help them to get active, and increase their bone density – just as I had been advised all those years ago.

Bones are very much alive, and change regularly: the breakdown of old tissue and the formation of fresh, new bone tissue keep them stable and healthy. During the middle-aged years, one of the key challenges is the risk of osteoporosis, a disease in which bones become thin and prone to fracture as they lose calcium and density. The menopause signifies the time when our reproductive systems are shutting down and our newly decreased oestrogen levels affect the rate at which new bone is formed. At sixty-five, about 30 per cent of women have osteoporosis, and nearly all of them are unaware of their condition. After age eighty, up to 70 per cent of women develop it.

Crucially, the condition of our skeletal frames depends on the peak bone density we reached prior to menopause and the rate at which you lose bone density after menopause. There are other factors such as genetics and dietary intake of calcium and vitamin D, which influence bone density but the main issue is oestrogen deficiency. Exercise is vital to bone strength, particularly load-bearing exercises such as weights and impact exercises such as running.[12]

Post-menopausal women are a staggering four times more likely to get osteoporosis than men. Scarily, they can lose 1 to 2 per cent of their bone mass annually – hence the importance of strength training to reduce the risk of fractures. One twelve-month study on post-menopausal women doing two days of strength training per week demonstrated 1 per cent gains in hip and spine bone density, 75 per cent increase in strength and 13 per cent increase in dynamic balance.[13] Although lower-intensity exercise (such as walking) is beneficial to bone density, higher-intensity exercise will have a more significant effect. Even for men, who don't have the complexities of the menopause, strength training is valuable. A study showed that men who ran nine or more times per month exhibited lower rates of lumbar bone loss than those who jogged less frequently.

One of the most common injuries for any older person is twisting an ankle, a mishap that often results from poor balance. If the ligament is damaged, then the neuro-receptors in the ligaments are also damaged, and the brain no longer gets reliable signals, meaning proprioception is impaired. Individuals become less stable and more prone to falling over again. A solution to poor balance is to practise just standing on one leg for two to three minutes on a stable – or, even better, a less stable – base. Or, ensuring suitable supports are nearby, you could try Silverfit's Tube surfing – balancing with no hands on the Underground or train, or on the bus. We test Silverfitters on how long they can balance on each leg – not to be competitive, but to give the individual the motivation to improve. Balance exercises such as tai chi are effective, or standing one-legged while waiting for a bus or cleaning your teeth.

Strength training also has an effect on other structures in the body: it improves the quality of the tissue and increases their load capacity. This applies equally to muscle fibres, tendons and cartilage. Muscles are either made up of endurance fibres, which are slow-twitch and contract slowly, or fast-twitch fibres, which contract quickly and vigorously. Older people need to retain those fast-twitch fibres to avoid potential falls.

Weight training is also the best protection against the loss of joint flexibility. Older people, indeed all adults, should also do resistance activities at a moderate or high intensity for all major muscle groups two or more days a week. This should include exercises for the chest, back, shoulders, thighs, hips, abdomen and lower legs. The exercises can be done with free weights, machines, resistance bands or simply with body weight.

Encouragingly, older women are recognised as being outstanding adherents to exercise programmes, particularly when exercising socially, so if women can be attracted to programmes of exercise within a more social context, there is clearly huge potential to help them to increase their fitness and feel in more control of their lives. Even more encouraging is another study on older women that found that outdoor workouts left women in a better mood and kept them exercising longer than counterparts who exercised indoors.[14]

There is a huge body of research concluding that the food we eat impacts on the risk of chronic disease.[15] The phrase 'we are what we eat' rings as true today as it did in my grandmother's time. Diet is believed to account for roughly 35 to 60 per cent of cancers, including cancers of the stomach, colon, liver, prostate, breast, uterus and ovary.[16] There is substantial agreement that a Mediterranean diet of fruit, vegetables, beans, whole grains, fish low in saturated fat and only small amount of dairy and meat leads to a reduction in obesity, high blood pressure, coronary heart disease, several cancers, diabetes, Alzheimer's disease and the risk of premature death.

Healthy diets not only help prevent cancer but evidence also suggests that they also reduce the risk of cancer re-occurring. A study followed nearly 2500 post-menopausal women with breast cancer for five years after treatment.[17] They found those who ate a diet full of fruit and vegetables, or exercised had less risk of re-occurrence of their cancer. If they ate fruit and veg and exercised, their risks were halved. A high-fibre diet is also related to decreased re-occurrence in women recently treated for breast cancer.[18] To summarise reports from the American cancer project, girls born now have a one in three risk of cancer, boys a one in two. Lifestyle factors such as smoking, exercise and diet are the major influences, not genetics. Meat-eaters with associated increased hormone levels have more colorectal cancer and those men eating dairy products a higher risk of prostate cancers.

Diet also has an influence on other conditions, such as Alzheimer's disease. An American study compared a group of 194 patients with Alzheimer's to 179 patients without any form of dementia and it was found that a higher adherence to the Mediterranean diet was associated with lower risk of Alzheimer's disease.[19]

Older adults eat on average 4.4 servings of fruit and vegetables daily, but only 37 per cent meet the national guidelines of five portions per day (compared with 30 per cent in younger age groups).[20] In a study of women in their seventies, those who were the most physically active and had the highest consumption of fruits and vegetables were eight times more likely to survive to the study's five-year follow-up than women with the lowest rates.[21]

Dietary protein is crucial for development of bone and muscle. Several epidemiological and clinical studies point to a beneficial effect of protein intakes above the current recommended daily allowance of 0.8 g/kg per day for adults aged nineteen and older – even as much as two grams of protein for every kilogram of body weight. However, nutritional studies show that many elderly individuals eat less protein than the average person, and there is also evidence that the muscles' response to dietary protein reduces with age. A diet containing a moderate amount of protein-rich food such as beef, fish, pork, chicken, dairy or nuts may help slow the deterioration of elderly people's muscles. Breakfast is a much-neglected meal in terms of protein intake, yet one scrambled egg and two veggie sausages provide thirty grams.[22]

Cholesterol (a lipid) is often seen as the enemy in the nutrition world, yet it is vital for the normal functioning of the body. It is mainly made by the liver, but can also be found in some foods. Having an excessively high level of lipids in your blood (hyperlipidaemia) can increase the risk of serious health conditions. But a cholesterol level is not in itself a good way to predict whether an individual will suffer from heart disease. There are other important risk factors, such as being overweight, smoking or a lack of exercise.

When I went for my free health check when I turned seventy, my cholesterol level was a little high and I fell within the band for whom statins could be prescribed. Not wanting to take a drug without understanding what it was for I went to do some more research. I found that statins, the medicines that can help lower rates of low-density lipoprotein (LDL) cholesterol (so-called bad cholesterol) in the blood, are the world's bestselling pharmaceutical drugs of all time. But the *British Medical Journal* has published a couple of articles documenting some of the side effects of statins, concluding that the dis-benefits may outweigh the benefits.[23] Another study I read, from Holland, asked 4738 statin users about side effects and of the quarter (27 per cent) who had suffered from them, 40 per cent experienced muscle pain, 31 per cent had joint pain, 16 per cent had digestion problems and 13 per cent had memory loss. I decided not to go on statins, although I am aware of recent research indicating they may have benefits for other conditions.

Looking back on the nutritional advice I have been given over the years, the one thing I have followed for fifty years is to take two tablespoonfuls of PLJ lemon juice in water first thing in the morning, along with a cod liver oil capsule. I figure that if the government insisted that, as kids in the forties, we needed cod liver oil, it must be good for us.

It isn't just our physical health that is impacted by exercise. In my fifty years of social work, and further consultancy work for Cooltan Arts, a mental health charity, I have seen a huge amount of evidence for the value of regular physical activity on psychological wellbeing, self-esteem, improved mental health and social integration. When centenarians and other long-lived individuals have been studied they attribute their longevity to healthy lifestyle, exercising regularly and – crucially – maintaining a social network and a positive mental attitude.[24]

The famous Marmot study found that three or more hours of average per day overtime of 10,308 civil servants led to stress and a 60 per cent increased risk of coronary heart disease.[25] Chronic stress, like depression, can lead to an increase in smoking, drinking, sedentary lifestyles and chronic inflammation, all of which have impact on the workplace and economy. Stress has huge effects on health but, with the right inspiration, motivation and support, exercise relieves stress, preventing the damaging chain reactions unleashed by the build-up of stress hormones.

Age UK carried out valuable research on an older group of people and found that when social wellbeing was introduced into the survey, older people said that wanted to exercise more. Interestingly, they also said they preferred to exercise in a group, even when they did not know the other people.

I never use the word lonely, and few of us oldies would ever admit it if we were. But in an ELSA study from 2012/13, Mark Hamer found that more than 1.32 million older men reported a moderate to high degree of social isolation and over seven hundred thousand reported a high degree of loneliness. The evidence also showed that older men were more isolated than older women. Sadly, 23 per cent of older men had less than monthly contact with their children, whereas for women that figure was only 15 per cent. But this doesn't surprise me; we seventy-plus oldies were the product of the sixties, when men went to work and women stayed at home to look after the kids. Very, very few of us went to university. Thank goodness for my enlightened father who, perhaps because he had no sons, assumed I would go. The lives of this generation of men were often work-based, and as a result 19 per cent of older men in the study had less than monthly contact with their friends. This contrasts with only 12 per cent of women. So if older men are more likely to be socially isolated, exercising with other oldies can be a vital lifeline for them. Reading Sir Muir Gray's inspirational and salutary book *Sod 70! – The Guide to Living Well* might help too.

While she was facing those long, long hours training for a marathon, the neuroscientist Leigh Leasure decided to study whether involuntary exercise had the same positive effect.[26] She set up an experiment with one group of mice running freely, another group trapped on a treadmill, and a third group remaining sedentary. After three weeks, the most new neurons appeared in the brains of mice that exercised voluntarily. She concluded that the study, although done in mice, could have implications for humans trying to exercise: 'Maybe what's important is for people to choose something they enjoy, not something that they are not really excited about doing and have to force themselves to engage in.'

Another great study Leasure ran was on sociable rats.[27] She found that rats with access to exercise wheels in their cages aged more healthily. However, when these rats were housed alone their brains did not benefit from exercise as much as when they shared cages. Socially housed rats, she found, produced copious amounts of new brain cells when they exercised; the lonely animals did not. It also seems that rats, like most runners I know, like a trip to the pub after exercise. Leasure found that exercising rats turned to alcohol with significantly more enthusiasm than sedentary rats, mainly during the first week of the experiment. 'It was a bit of a surprise,' Dr Leasure said. From my experience of fellow exercise junkies, I was less surprised.

While social isolation can be combated through exercise, so too can more serious mental health issues. A recent study found that uncontrolled high blood pressure and diabetes contribute to the loss of brain cells.[28] Aerobic exercise protects the brain by building heart and artery resilience, which boosts blood flow to the brain. Dr Noel Collins, an older-adult psychiatrist specialising in ageing population and a fellow

Serpentine runner, says that there is emerging evidence of significant psychological and cognitive benefits from regular exercise reducing the risk of dementia. He cited an important multinational three-year European study that included annual full cognitive assessments of 639 people in their sixties and seventies. Researchers found older people who engage in regular physical activity reduced their risk of vascular-related dementia by 40 per cent and cognitive impairment by 60 per cent.[29] In a large study, 1740 people older than sixty-five and with no cognitive impairment were followed biennially to identify the presence of dementia. After six years 158 participants had developed dementia and 107 had developed Alzheimer's. Analysis found that regular exercise was associated with a delay in the onset of both dementia and Alzheimer's disease.[30]

Dr Collins adds, 'There is now compelling evidence that staying active – physically, mentally and socially – is the key to maintaining good health and quality of life as we age. I have told this to hundreds of patents in my memory clinic, explaining that remaining active in mind and body can help delay the onset or progression of dementia. Any activity that manages to combine physical, social and intellectual elements, such as a Silverfit walking group that gets the blood and the conversation going in people, is bound to have dramatic benefit over time. My only wish is that I could pre-scribe activity as readily as medication to my patients. I also hope that more research into the benefit of activity will be conducted and the results will encourage millions of people to remain active at every age. If this occurs, I imagine that future doctors will have considerably fewer older patients sitting in their waiting rooms.'

An Australian research group analysed thirty-nine studies relating to physical activity and delayed cognitive decline and concluded that physical exercise improved cognitive function in the over-fifties. The report went on to recommend both aerobic and resistance exercise of at least moderate intensity on as many days of the week as possible.[31] Exercise keeps the mind sharp. The theory is that, through exercise, the brain receives a greater supply of blood, oxygen and nutrients that boost brain health, as well as the growth hormone that helps the formation of new neurons (neurogenesis) and connections.

So why does this happen? Pioneering animal studies have shown that the brains of athletic mice showed two to three times more neurogenesis than the non-exerciser mice. Subsequent research into the human brain has showed that it is not only capable of renewing itself, but that exercise speeds the process.

Mitochondria is not a word that many of us come across on a day-to-day basis, yet these tiny organelles generate the energy that our cells need to do their jobs. Mitochondria are defined as the powerhouse of the cells. They convert food fuel into forms that can be used by muscles. When a muscle starts to move, mitochondria within the muscle cells use either the sugar in the muscles (glycogen) or the sugars in the bloodstream to make ATP (adenosine triphosphate), a specialised molecule that provides energy to contracting muscles. Increased numbers of mitochondria means an increase in the rate of energy production. In turn, muscles, bones and ligaments become stronger to cope with the additional stresses and impact put through them.

Over time, as we age, mutations begin to outstrip our system's ability to make repairs and mitochondria start malfunctioning and dying. As resident mitochondria falter, the cells they fuel wither or die. Muscles shrink, brain volume drops, and hair falls out or loses its pigmentation. All too soon, both in appearance and beneath the surface, we are old. The more mitochondria you have, the more energy you can generate during exercise and the faster and longer you can exercise. Is it significant that my grey hair, whilst rather red (courtesy of Clairol), is still strong and wiry?

Again, many of the interesting studies have been done on mice. In a famous and influential experiment, Dr Mark Tarnopolsky's mice were bred so that they lacked the normal mitochondrial repair mechanism. This meant 'they developed malfunctioning mitochondria early in their lives, as early as three months of age, the human equivalent of age twenty. By the time they reached eight months, or their early six-ties in human terms, the animals were extremely frail and decrepit, with spindly muscles, shrunken brains, enlarged hearts, shrivelled gonads and patchy, graying fur. Listless, they barely moved around their cages. All were dead before reaching a year of age.' But, fascinatingly, this was not true for the mice that exercised. At eight months, Dr Tarnopolsky reports that 'when their sedentary lab mates were bald, frail and dying, the running rats remained youthful. They had full pelts of dark fur, no salt-and-pepper shadings. They also had maintained almost all of their muscle mass and brain volume. Their gonads were normal, as were their hearts.'[32] They could even balance on narrow rods – the show-offs, as he described them.

In a human study, researchers found that, in both men and women with an average age of sixty-seven, regular exercise significantly increased mitochondrial content, indicating that exercise is a realistic and practical way to increase energy and endurance in both younger and older adults.

Like mitochondria, telomeres are also something else we are unlikely to consider very often, yet they have a huge impact on how we age.

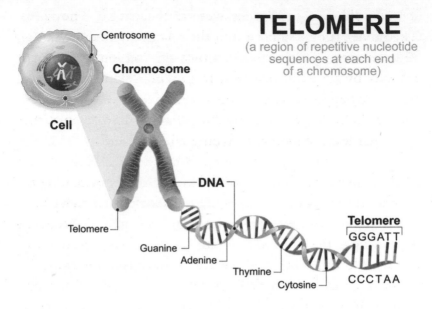

Telomeres are tiny chromosomes (the protective caps) on the ends of DNA strands. When cells divide and replicate these long strands of DNA, the telomere cap is snipped, a process that is believed to protect the rest of the DNA but leaves an increasingly abbreviated telomere. Eventually, if a cell's telomeres become too short, the cell either dies or enters a kind of suspended state. That is ageing. Most researchers now accept telomere length as a reliable marker of cell age, and thus health.

Fortunately, there are many ways people can prevent and reduce shortened telomeres, including taking steps to reduce chronic stress and work-related exhaustion, improving diet (a December 2012 study found the Mediterranean diet to be protective), minimising exposure to air pollution, exercising consistently, moderating alcohol consumption and viewing stressful situations as challenges instead of threats.

When researchers measured telomeres, sedentary older subjects had telomeres that were on average 40 per cent shorter than in the sedentary young subjects, suggesting

that the older subjects' cells were also ageing.[33] They also
tested older runners and found they had remarkably youthful telomeres: a bit shorter than those in the young runners,
but only by about 10 per cent. In general, telomere loss was
reduced by approximately 75 per cent in the ageing runners,
leading the researchers to conclude that exercise, even at the
molecular level, has an anti-ageing effect.

Finally, sleep. Sleep is a vital physiological process with
important restorative functions. But notable qualitative and
quantitative changes in sleep occur with age. Moreover,
many sleep-related disorders occur with increasing frequency
among elderly people, and we are becoming more aware of
the adverse impact on sleep of blue light, associated with using
our phones, tablets and TVs in the last hour or so before bed.
    People who exercise regularly enjoy improved sleep quality,
they fall asleep more easily, wake less often and sleep longer.
We know severe sleep disturbances may lead to depression,
cognitive impairments, deterioration of quality of life and
significant stresses for carers and increased healthcare costs.
The most common treatment for sleep disorders (particularly
insomnia) is drugs. But yet again there is some evidence that
physical exercise, taken regularly, may promote relaxation
and raise core body temperature in ways that are beneficial
to initiating and maintaining sleep. Happily, I sink into bed
and sleep brilliantly, awoken abruptly by an alarm telling me
it is time to go swimming, cycling or running!

Notes to chapter 12

1   See <http://www.elsa-project.ac.uk/>.
2   Steve C. Moore et al., 'Leisure Time Physical Activity of Moderate to
    Vigorous Intensity and Mortality: A Large Pooled Cohort Analysis',
    PLoS Medicine, 9:11 (2012).

3   Agency for Healthcare Research and Quality; Centres for Disease
    Control and Prevention, 'Physical Activity and Older Americans:
    Benefits and Strategies', June 2002; and M. Pratt, C. A. Macera and G.
    Wang, 'Higher direct medical costs associated with physical inactivity',
    The Physician and Sportsmedicine, 28:10 (2000), 63–70.

4   Baohui Zhang et al., 'Health Care Costs in the Last Week of Life:
    Associations with End of Life Conversations', *Archives of Internal Medicine*,
    169:5 (2009), 480–8.

5   J. Stessman et al., 'Physical activity, function, and longevity among the
    very old', *Archives of Internal Medicine*, 169:16 (2009), 1476–83.

6   Quoted in Gretchen Reynolds, *The First 20 Minutes: The Surprising
    Science of How We Can Exercise Better, Train Smarter, Live Longer* (New
    York: Hudson Street Press, 2012).

7   Fiona F. Stanway et al., 'How fast does the Grim Reaper walk? Receiver
    operating characteristics curve analysis in healthy men aged 70 and
    over', *British Medical Journal*, 343 (2011).

8   See 'Case study': Beat the Street: getting communities moving', Public
    Health England, 19 July 2016, <https://www.gov.uk/government/
    case-studies/beat-the-street-getting-communities-moving>.

9   Jennifer Abbasi, 'Strength training helps older adults live longer', Penn
    State Vice President for Research website, <https://www.research.psu.
    edu/node/383>.

10 'Hospital inpatient care: almost 900 more admissions per day
    compared to previous year', NHS Digital, 25 February 2015,
    <http://content.digital.nhs.uk/article/6053/Hospital-inpatient-care-
    almost-900-more-admissions-per-day-compared-to-previous-
    year>.

11 Lisa Rapaport, 'Tai chi tied to reduced fall risk in older adults',
    Reuters Health, 17 February 2017, <http://www.reuters.com/article/
    us-health-tai-chi-fall-prevention-idUSKBN15W24Z>.

12 Ian Murnaghan, 'Menopause and Bone Health', Menopause Expert
    website, <http://www.menopauseexpert.co.uk/menopause-bone-
    health.html>.

13 http://growingstronger.nutrition.tufts.edu/why_grow_stronger/
    research_and_background.html.

14 Shereen Lehman, 'Older Women Who Exercise Outdoors More Likely
    to Stick with It', *Scientific American*, <https://www.scientificamerican.
    com/article/older-women-who-exercise-outdoors-more-
    likely-to-stick-with-it/>.

15 A. F. Kramer, K. I. Erickson and S. J. Colcombe, 'Exercise, cognition,
    and the aging brain', *Journal of Applied Physiology*, 10:4 (2006),
    1237–42.

16 See www.cancerproject.org and http://www.cancerproject.org/.

17 Cited in N. D. Barnard and J. K. Reilly, *The Cancer Survivor's Guide:*

Foods That Help You Fight Back (Summertown: Healthy Living Publications, 2008), p. 48.

18 E. B. Gold et al., 'Dietary factors and vasomotor symptoms in breast cancer survivors: the WHEL Study', *Menopause*, 13:3 (2006), 423–33.

19 Nikolaos Scarmeas et al., 'Mediterranean Diet, Alzheimer Disease, and Vascular Mediation', *Archives of Neurology*, 63:2 (2006), 1709–17.

20 Department of Health, 'Statistical Press Notice: National Diet and Nutrition Survey: headline results from years 1, 2 and 3 combined (2008/09 – 2010/11)', 25 July 2012.

21 E. J. Nicklett et al., 'Fruit and vegetable intake, physical activity, and mortality in older community-dwelling women', *Journal of the American Geriatric Society*, 60:5 (2012), 862–8.

22 Denise Webb, 'Protein for Fitness: Age Demands Greater Protein Needs', *Today's Dietician*, 17:4 (2015), 16, <http://www.todaysdietitian. com/newarchives/040715p16.shtml>.

23 See J. D. Abramson et al., 'Should people at low risk of cardiovascular disease take a statin?', *BMJ*, 347 (2013); and A. Malhotra, 'Saturated fat is not the major issue', *BMJ*, 347 (2013).

24 T. E. Seeman et al., 'Behavioral and psychosocial predictors of physical performance: MacArthur studies of successful aging', *Journals of Gerontology: Series A – Biological Sciences and Medical Sciences*, 50:4 (1995), 177–83. Waneen Spirduso, Karen Francis and Priscilla MacRae, *Physical Dimensions of Aging* (Champaign: Human Kinetics, 2005).

25 M. Marmot et al., 'Health inequalities among British civil servants: the Whitehall II study', *Lancet*, 337:8754 (1991), 1387–93, <http://www. thelancet.com/journals/lancet/article/PII0140-6736(91)93068-K/ abstract?cc=y=>.

26 J. L. Leasure, 'Forced and voluntary exercise differentially affect brain and behavior', *Neuroscience*, 156:3 (2008), 456–65.

27 M. E. Maynard and J. L. Leasure, 'Exercise enhances recovery following binge ethanol exposure', *PLoS One*, 8:9 (2013).

28 L. D. Baker et al., 'Effects of aerobic exercise on mild cognitive impairment: a controlled trial', *Archives of Neurology*, 67:1 (2010), 71–9.

29 A. Verdelho et al., 'Physical Activity Prevents Progression for Cognitive Impairment and Vascular Dementia Results from the LADIS (Leukoaraiosis and Disability) Study', *Stroke*, 43 (2012), 3331–5.

30 E. B. Larson et al., 'Exercise Is Associated with Reduced Risk for Incident Dementia among Persons 65 Years of Age and Older', *Annals of Internal Medicine*, 144:2 (2006), 73–81.

31 Joseph Michael Northey et al., 'Exercise interventions for cognitive function in adults older than 50: a systematic review with meta-analysis', *British Journal of Sports Medicine* (2017), <http://dx.doi.org/10.1136/ bjsports-2016-096587>.

32 Gretchen Reynolds, 'Can Exercise Keep You Young?', *New York*

Times, 2 March 2011. See also Meredith Melnick, 'Study: Can Exercise Keep Us from Aging', *Time*, 3 Mary 2011, <http://healthland.time.com/2011/03/03/study-can-exercise-keep-us-from-aging/>.

33   Cited in Reynolds, *The First 20 Minutes*.

13

Coping with adversity and failure

Working long, long voluntary hours on Silverfit, with even less time to train, I questioned how I came to sign up for Ironman Lanzarote again in 2015. Its reputation was as the toughest in the world. Was it because Steve was also doing it, or that I had so loved the 2013 experience, with all those friends around me in such a beautifully scenic place? Was it the happy memories of our annual Serpentine trip to Club La Santa? Or was it another challenge for an older woman unwilling or unable to accept the normal ageing process when my sons were jocularly suggesting I should get back to knitting and start watching the TV.

In reality, it was just one of those serendipitous happenings. At the race in Hyde Park in 2013, when the BBC had followed my training and the race, I had also qualified to be a member of the age-group team for the World Triathlon Championships in Edmonton, Canada, the following year. Annie was giving me regular programmes focused on the shorter Olympic distance. I have always found those workouts more challenging – reaching and sustaining a higher pain level in high-intensity workouts. I am really much happier doing the long, slow stuff. Looking at my diary for Silverfit and taking into account the high cost of the trip to Canada, I was hesitating.

I rang Annie, and left a voicemail: 'Annie, I am having second thoughts about the Edmonton trip. I am just not sure I want to go. You know what? I think I might even prefer to do another Ironman in Lanzarote.' Annie must have picked up the message right away as no sooner had I put the phone down than she had told the world via her extensive social media links that this old woman was going to do another Ironman Lanzarote. Such is the power of social media that my friend Isabelle, who worked at Club La Santa, picked up on Annie's Facebook and Twitter messages and blasted it out even further. The following morning I realised that if so many people thought I was going to do it, I had better sign up.

I had even less time than in the previous year to put in the mileage on the bike. However, with profound thanks to the leisure providers GLL/Better, I had been awarded one of their GLL Foundation Awards, which gave me free access to all their facilities, and in particular their spin classes. I love spinning, so I packed in loads of sessions at Brixton Recreation Centre. My Thursday and Friday evenings were often spent in hard double sessions with instructors Sara, Sheila or Imla. Those ninety minutes would have me standing on the bike for most of the time, pedalling against hard gears, only sitting back on the saddle occasionally, and then to spin as fast as possible. The hours spent in the standing position would stand me in great stead in the year to come. But, for me, the greatest motivator for sticking to it was pedalling to the fabulous house, garage and reggae music late into the evening. I was always the oldest in the group, but it was such a friendly and welcoming and fun environment.

Following the spin sessions, at around 9 p.m., I would get into the almost empty 25-metre pool. Most normal people probably had far better options than swimming for spending their evening in Brixton. After my swim I'd go home, past POP BRIXTON, that innovative shipping container village that our Silverfit cheerleaders had helped to launch, past the buzzing bars, the fantastic night market, and finally down the escalator at Brixton Underground. With just a tinge of envy, I would watch the hordes of young, bubbly, happy people coming upwards to the nightlife that Brixton has to offer. I rationalised it, saying to myself, 'No alcohol for me tonight, I must be ready to train early tomorrow morning.' But it would have been fun to join them.

Thanks to Freedom Sports, I had been given a really generous discount to buy a new DeVinci bike – one that might get me up the hills just a bit faster. A Canadian manufacturer, making our rental bikes in London, I understood this was one of their first women's road bikes being sold in the UK. I loved the new bike and it fitted perfectly. I knew I would need all the help I could get. The annual Serpentine trip to Lanzarote in March gave me some serious bike miles, and I was able to join part of a swim training camp run by Swim for Tri over at Club La Santa too. Unfortunately, there was no time to get out to Cesenatico. I did some Parkruns in my local, friendly venue, one of the best Parkrun venues for personal-best times, Burgess Park, and occasionally a longer run, still trying to minimise the pressure on my knees. Unforgivably, I struggled to fit in Elaine's recommendations for stretching and strength building.

Surely, I told myself, Lanzarote couldn't be as windy as it had been in 2013. How wrong I was. It really was very, very windy, and we knew from the outset the bike ride would be tough. I realised too that there was a new cut-off time on the bike, towards the end of the climbs in the north of the island. If I didn't make the aid station at Haría by a specific time, I would not be allowed to continue, as the roads would be re-opened to traffic.

The first swim lap felt fine, but after getting back up onto the sand bank I glanced at my watch before plunging back into the water. It had taken over an hour. I was surprised I had been that much slower than two years earlier. Maybe this was because there were fewer people on the second lap or maybe, as I concluded later, the swell really did build up. It was really, really hard going. I vividly remember swimming just after the 3k turn point, on the second lap, and looking down at a rock below. Ten hard strokes later, and hard kicking, and that small rock was still below me. It was little wonder that I got cramp for the first time ever on a swim. I had no idea how to counteract it – there was nothing solid to stretch out against. I knew that I could just put my hand up and a canoeist would come rushing over to my rescue. Should I, or shouldn't I? Could I give up? If I did, it would be the end of my race. Finally, I just lay in the water and relaxed, the cramp eased and I swam slowly back to the exit point. I emerged with the commentator and the crowds cheering me on. I had just, and only just, made the swim cut-off of 2 hours, 20 minutes. I was exhausted but overjoyed. Back in transition there were still far more bikes there than I usually saw. I hadn't been the last out of the water and many hadn't made the swim cut-off. The bike leg, I reassured myself, would be fun.

It wasn't. It was very hard. I watched my average speed drop and drop further, even around the awesome El Golfo loop, where I was usually on a real high along that fabulous undulating coastal route, with huge waves dashing against the black volcanic rock. I passed a few fellow cyclists and then, after about 30k, a police car overtook me, waved and then went back to follow me. It was a while before the penny dropped. I must be the last cyclist; those behind me had pulled out.

Having a police escort induces an embarrassing yet reassuring feeling. Other cars only overtook the police and me when it was really safe to do so. Oncoming cars slowed down before cautiously going past. The policemen marshalling at junctions were especially enthusiastic as we went by and they saw my police escort. Going up that long hill to Fire Mountain into the wind was so hard, and at the top I managed, just, to turn and wave to my companions, before hurtling down the other side. I was having such fun and I really wanted to chat to them, but it wasn't an option. Finally, after 40k or so, I overtook another cyclist, and with a short beep of the horn, I lost my personal bodyguards. Thanks, guys.

At 100k I could see I wasn't going to make the cut-off time, although I did wonder if they would extend it given the high winds. I overtook another guy who was struggling. We both knew we wouldn't make it and together we stopped at a loo station, about 2k short of the formal cut-off point. There were five of us, and thankfully we got into a truck, with our bikes dumped in behind us. It was with mixed emotions that we were going down from the mountains in the truck. I was frustrated to be missing out on that wonderful descent on the bike, where the wind would be so powerfully behind me. But again the camaraderie and humour made defeat bearable. Four of us joked that at least we didn't have to do the marathon. The fifth guy, inexplicably to me, seemed determined to do it once we got back to Puerto del Carmen, even though he wouldn't get a real time.

Back into town, we were now there to support other competitors who were out on the run. Within minutes I saw Steve coming up to the turnaround before going out on his final lap. I guess he felt a mixture of relief and sadness to see his mother, safe and sound yet clearly not to be an Ironman finisher. It had been a hard, hard day.

Steve has never been one to wear his finisher's T-shirts, apart from at the customary 'morning after the Ironman' breakfast. But not so in 2015. The next time we all went out for a drink in his local pub in London, there he was, Ironman Lanzarote 2015: FINISHER. Nothing like rubbing salt in the wound. I love my kids!

Back home it took me a while to recover and reflect on my failure, and the lack of a finisher's T-shirt – despite the fact that I knew three hundred other people hadn't made it either. Reassuring statements like 'It wasn't failure: you did 100k' meant little. Always needing a goal, I wondered what would be my next one. I started to read more about sports stars who had had to cope with their failure in a far more public way, and realised it was often about an inner resilience and, even more importantly, confidence.

Should I sign up for 2016, or just do the half distance of 70.3 miles next time? Or maybe, just maybe, another, less wind-affected Ironman? I wondered if seventy-two-year-old bodies were really made for two Ironman distances in a year. Endlessly, I debated within myself. I hadn't put myself through the marathon in Lanzarote, so perhaps, I reassured myself, it didn't really count as a full Ironman. After a few weeks of this and so many of my friends asking 'What next?' came the real clincher. Steve was already signed up for Ironman Vichy at the end of August and he offered to drive my bike down there, whilst I relaxed on the Eurostar. What a star. The swim would be in a lake and the bike route, we thought, was fairly flat. Annie didn't hesitate: 'Go for it, you can do it!' Or maybe it was the influence of 'This Girl Can!' The campaign to get more women more active had been very successful and both the Gym Group, who had awarded me life membership, and British Triathlon were about to feature me in their monthly magazines. Could I really say to them 'This girl can't?' Nothing like pressure, so Vichy Ironman it was to be.

There was also another goal, of finishing the New York Triathlon to come. This year both sons, my son-in-law and my adopted son Chris were all determined to beat my winning swim split of the previous year. All four steered a better course towards the centre of the river, and left me in fifth place. But it was great fun. How fortunate to have such an opportunity for shared family fun and celebratory drinks afterwards. This year, though, the drinks were a bit curtailed as I left that same evening to get back to London for the following night's *Independent on Sunday* 'Happy 100' party celebrating those who make Britain a happier place to live.

It was an incredible privilege to be one of the hundred people selected for that award. A Serpie friend, Dan Bent, was also one of the Happy 100. He had set up Project Awesome with the objective of promoting free opportunities for exercise and fun together in a variety of park venues. After the formal event we celebrated late into the night, along with the inspirational Annie Ross. Annie, an active travel writer, adventure enthusiast and *Evening Standard* online journalist, had set up Exerkyourself to encourage others to a more active lifestyle. But she had also completed a mind-blowing fifty-two sporting challenges in fifty-two weeks. She organised a race one evening around the Circle line on the Underground, for which Silverfit entered a relay team. We loved the experience.

As ideal training for Vichy, Annie Emmerson and I scheduled a couple of long bike rides. First came the Prudential RideLondon hundred-miler, by now in its third year and with up to thirty thousand riders taking part. The weather was dry and warm – a massive contrast to the dire conditions of the previous year – so hopefully there was the possibility of actually being able to climb Leith Hill. However, even in dry weather I thought that climb up the second-highest hill in southern England was risky with such a large number of riders. Narrow at one of the steepest parts, in the first year, in 2012, there were riders walking up the hill on the left hand side, others, like me, struggling in the middle, and faster riders on the right weaving their way in and out of us slower riders as they overtook us, to gain time and distance. Leith Hill had felt like an accident waiting to happen. On the descent, paramedics were giving first aid after two crashes.

This year, though, it was a sad, sad occasion that closed the Leith Hill climb. Despite very speedy medical attention and a helicopter rescue service, a fifty-five-year-old man had collapsed and died at the scene. It wasn't an accident or colliding bikes, but one of those awful life incidents that leaves you reflecting that stuff happens. I had been profoundly moved when I heard Dr Hugh Montgomery, the director of the Institute for Human and Health and Performance at UCL, on *Desert Island Discs* in 2014, and his words have never left me. He had said, in that memorable interview, 'You never know what's around the corner. Enjoy life while you can.'

I also loved the Allianz Surrey Classic hundred-mile ride, held a couple of weeks later in the same region but with different climbs in those beautiful Surrey Hills, and with great signage all the way so that you didn't have to keep stopping to look at a map or a phone – knowing, too, that every 20k or so there would be a few welcoming faces and a refreshments station. With most riders probably by now having completed the ride and back at base, I always feel guilty if I am one of the last; these poor volunteers at aid and refreshment posts have had to hang around for just a few of us, but they are always so gracious.

With perfect timing, three weeks before the Ironman, I was signed up for the longer 80k bike ride in the London Triathlon, along with the shorter Olympic distance 1.5k swim and run. For me, it was only going to be training event: nothing hardcore before Vichy. The swim was fine. I had hoped for the magical, longer bike route past the Tower of London, along the Embankment and down to Big Ben but instead it was four 20k laps, with a fiddly bit up and around Canary Wharf that was a real challenge. As I came down the last few kilometres of the penultimate lap, I could feel my saddle had moved back a tiny bit. Foolishly, I wasn't carrying my toolkit. In vain, I looked out for a mechanic on the route who could maybe tighten the screw a bit. I was used to a number of bike mechanics and support vehicles on an Ironman course, so was dismayed not to see one. There were ambulances and first aiders at key points but not a mechanic in sight.

Suddenly, in Canary Wharf, my seat post collapsed completely. I could no longer sit down on the saddle, which was at right-angles to the bike. I still had 14k to go. I went down into the Limehouse tunnel, up again and around the turn-point, and back down and up again. Well, I figured, if I can do that one kilometre distance and the tunnel gradients standing up all the time, then maybe, just maybe, I could get to the end. I visualised the spin sessions I did with Imla, Sheila and Sarah, imagining the beat of the house and garage music, and all those hours spent at Brixton Rec and Sarah's command to 'stand tall, bum back towards the saddle, up again, press left shoulder down towards the right, right shoulder to the left, back upright, move the bum side to side, down to the left, down to the right, crouch back'.

I sailed past ExCeL and into the last 5k. Crouching low and backwards whenever I could and pulling my abs in as my spin instructors insisted, I might just be able to make it. Down the final mile, I was going to make it. I was triumphant. The slope up to ExCeL was really hard work for my exhausted muscles. The official at the top instructed me rather firmly to 'Dismount NOW!' as I went over the white line and the timing mat. I wasn't at all sure I could get my shattered legs up and over the crossbar. He looked on in astonishment as I showed him my saddle precariously perched at that odd angle on the broken seat post.

And then the final dilemma as I walk/jogged the long transition to deposit my bike, wondering if, with all that pressure on my abs, hamstrings, quads and glutes, I would be able to walk, let alone run. I could see both sons having fun at my expense for not even attempting the run. I could hear them teasing: 'This Old Woman Can't!' I figured, too, that I really needed the experience of shattered biking muscles and then getting out onto a long run. I hadn't had to do that in Lanzarote but I would in Vichy. I staggered out, the only person walking rather than jogging the first four hundred metres, down a slope that my knees never like anyway, and then out along the three-lap run. I managed in the end to walk/run gently, and just get round. On the run back into ExCeL, as I approached the last five hundred metres of the race, a lovely DJ on the Bose stand managed to find 'Don't Stop Me Now'. His timing was absolutely perfect – as I passed, Queen were reaching their crescendo. He had also worked the crowd up as I'd gone back up the slope for the last lap, and Steve Trew, the commentator, was telling everyone of my twenty-seven years of age – 'Oh no, I think I may have that number back to front,' he added.

*

Vichy is a beautiful city, but a forthcoming Ironman tends to mean you are not in the mood for sightseeing, even though the thermal baths and museum are on the doorstep. It had been great to travel without having to lug a bike box, to be able to sit down peacefully on the train, writing fund-raising bids for Silverfit, while Steve drove my bike down through France.

The half-distance Ironman 70.3 was on the Saturday and the full Ironman on the Sunday. Coincidentally, my GP was out there for the weekend, supporting her partner doing the 70.3. Francesca, another friend and one of our Silverfit Nordic walking instructors, was doing the 70.3 too, so on the Saturday I got up early to watch her 70.3 swim start with her husband and support her and other athletes on the run, reflecting that it was a good way to relax and distract myself from the race the following day. With the main event area over on the other side of the lake, I spent many hours walking around it, or just gazing at the beauty and the movement of the water, incredibly worried about my ability to swim 3.8k albeit with the newfound confidence of a smaller wetsuit – thanks to Dan, Swim for Tri and Speedo – that actually fitted me properly rather than having the masses of empty space inside my older wetsuit that tended to fill up with water, or which had, like the orange-finned one, far too many holes in the neoprene – a consequence of gel nails pulling wetsuits off and on!

On Saturday evening, at the pasta party, we sat in long, long rows with a huge screen and commentators talking to us from the platform in front. I was happily chatting when I glanced at the big screen and suddenly saw my name up there. I have forgotten much of my school French, but could see they were celebrating the oldest and youngest competitors. The youngest, twenty-one-year-old James Tufnell, was already getting up onto the platform and they were looking round for me. I kept my head down for thirty seconds and then, nudged by Steve, I stood up and went onto the platform. It was a lovely idea, the oldest and the youngest, with James committing publicly to wait around for me at the end until I came in. I told him it would be a long wait. It is such a humbling experience when us oldies are given such incredibly positive support and acclamation: a roomful of supporters standing up to cheer – great athletes later wanting selfies with me as the oldie. However, it does add to the pressure as they will want me to finish too. Sadly, James was forced to pull out, with severe cramp, and get medical assistance.

My major anxiety was just beginning to surface: the water temperature. If it went above 24° Celsius then it would be decreed a non-wetsuit swim. Having gained confidence from my new wetsuit, and knowing it gave my heavy legs the buoyancy I sorely needed, I was very worried – to the point of doubting whether I would and could do the race without it. The water temperature on the Saturday was right on the cusp. A clear night or a cloudy sky might yet make that crucial difference.

Race morning dawned and, after the usual silent breakfast at some ungodly hour, a taxi arrived to take a few of us around the lake to the start point. Did anyone, I was asking myself, not feel the same level of panic I was feeling? The 70.3 the day before had been a wetsuit-legal swim, but whilst I doubted my ability to even complete 3.8k without a wetsuit, I guess the majority were far more worried about their swim time and the washing machine effect. At least, I didn't have to worry about that, I thought. I was fairly sure I could improve on my 2:19 swim time from Lanzarote in May, just one minute inside the cut-off time, if I could wear a wetsuit.

As the sun came up, we arrived at the transition area and I

caught sight of that unbelievably welcome noticeboard – the water temperature was 23.6° C. Now that was a very close call. I decided I would have to enjoy the swim now. With my wetsuit happily pulled on and goggles secure, I went down to the start gantry where it was time for the red hats of my wave to get into the water and swim to the start point. Another countdown, a few enthusiastic shouts and we were off. Although safe and well-marked, calm and with minimal current or wind, the swim in a murky lake lacked the joy of a sea swim and watching the fish below. It was a strange experience, finishing the first 1.9k, clambering up the ramp, under the gantry, making right turn, and back onto another jetty. Most jumped, a few dived, but I sat down on the edge. Francesca was now supporting me and her husband who was competing. She says she watched me sitting down for ages on the edge. She had wondered anxiously if I was going to withdraw from the race again, so she shouted 'Get back in the water!' I finally plopped into the lake again, for another 1.9k!

I had so looked forward to the two laps of 90k on the bike, with what I thought would be clear roads and woodland, but actually the bike section was really tough. The wind built up, and it was hot, very hot: an average of 36° C the whole time. Muscles I didn't know existed were cramping and I found myself having to rise out of the saddle to gain some relief. Maybe after my experience at the London Triathlon three weeks earlier, my glutes were a bit stronger. They really needed to be, as I found myself standing more and more to ease the cramp. I was so glad I had bought a bag of salted peanuts and chickpeas the previous day, and could pick at them – the salt eased the cramp. There was nothing salty on offer at the bike aid stations, so I eked out my meagre provisions. Later, a woman in the changing tent told me she had resorted to sucking her hair for the salt in her sweat. As

we passed through one village, a guy was offering to throw
a bowl of cold water over cyclists as they passed. I gratefully accepted, closed my eyes, and welcomed the shock to
the system.

What struck me most was the huge number of marshals –
three to four of them at every junction, and there were an
unusually high number of junctions leading onto our main-
road route, which was closed to traffic. The marshals were
patiently re-directing any vehicle trying to get out onto the
main road. Although most of them were still managing to
encourage each rider, I was aware that they had probably been
out in the high temperature, many with no shade around,
for eight or nine hours. They must have been absolutely
shattered.

I also saw more medics out on the route than usual and
people lying at the roadside, clearly exhausted, cramping or
dehydrated. Over the last 30k, I didn't want to push it too
hard, but was increasingly worried about the 5.30 p.m. cut-
off for the bike. I calculated that if I kept going, I would just
about make it, but it was very hard and I was shattered. But
if I am honest, I also knew that if I met that key deadline of
5.30 p.m., and completed the marathon part of the Ironman,
then Silverfit, with our key message of getting inactive oldies
more active, would benefit. The media would like the story of
a seventy-two-year-old completing an Ironman and encouraging other older people. So finally, I was cycling down the
steep hill into Vichy and back towards transition. I had fifteen
minutes to spare.

Suddenly, as I was finishing the bike course, there was my
son Steve running parallel to me on the run course. I would
happily have stopped for a chat, but although he was clearly
relieved to see me he was on a mission. At the end of the bike
I doubted I could even swing my right leg over my saddle to

get off. I was so stiff. As I slowly walked through transition my leg muscles were cramping badly. I steadied myself and stretched my leg against a paramedic, then a van driver, and then even a policeman, all of whom were encouraging me to seek medical help and pull out. I longed to give up, but reflected that the Ironman timings give a generous allowance for the marathon. A walk/run was possible within the six hours that still remained. Mind games again.

I set off walking, for at least the first kilometre, hoping the cramp would ease and, miraculously, it did. Gently I tried the odd hundred metres of jogging, counting up as I always do to fifty steps, then maybe a hundred steps, and then I could give myself permission to walk again. What amazed me was the number of other runners, their yellow wristbands denoting they were on their fourth and final lap, all walking. It was reassuring that it wasn't just my old woman's body that had been depleted by the heat and the effort.

It is a lovely run course – around the lake, deep into a wood and then up into the city for a short interlude. The support was fantastic. With a race number and EDWINA clearly printed on my tri-suit, the support was often individualised with many people calling my name. Then suddenly out at the far point I heard a fantastically motivating 'EDDIE! Go, go, and go!' It was from Lesley, another friend. She and her husband, John Levison of Tri 247, were there watching my last two laps. When I had doubted my own ability to finish yet another lap in time, it was just the encouragement I needed.

The sunset over the lake was fabulous. The route curved back though the crowds in the main finishing arena and then there was a left turn for another lap or the right lane to finish. How envious was I of those finishers, when I still had 30k to go. The commentators saw me and rabble-roused the crowd to support their seventy-two-year-old competitor. Then

I was back onto the run route again, away from the noise and the lights and into the peace of the course, the runners reducing dramatically as time went on. Oh how I wanted a yellow band and the sensation of being on the last lap. As it darkened, I asked about light in the woods, and on my third lap the volunteers offered me a glow-in-the-dark wristband.

I went back into the arena for the penultimate time. Anxiously, I asked the commentators if they thought I could make it before the cut-off. 'GO, GO, and GO!' they shouted at me. So off into the dark I jogged, for the final lap.

By 10 p.m. there were very few runners left out on the route. Most of the pathways were fine, with good paved surfaces and lighting, except that beautiful soft ground of the wood. In the wood it was absolutely pitch black – no lighting, no marshals, no runners to follow, and no clear path across the tree roots and other potential obstacles. It was scary and all too easy to get lost. But after a few deviations, I was back out into the light for the final push for home, with the disco at the end. Just 2k to run. The need to make the cut-off and to see the fireworks at 11.30 was my driving force.

By 11.19, I had made it. My total time was 16 hours and 6 minutes. The crowd in the arena were being worked up for all the final few finishers like me. They Mexican-waved me around that final loop and – this time – down the finishing straight. Words can't describe my feelings of ecstasy, euphoria, exhaustion and total relief. What a proud mum too, to have Steve, who had finished over three hours before me, waiting at the finish line, at least a drink or two ahead of me! Life was fun, my family so, so supportive. How effective could I be in 2016 promoting heathier ageing, and prevention of all those chronic diseases linked to inactivity, and a sedentary lifestyle backed so strongly by junk food and drink?

14

Onwards and upwards

2016 and 2017 were fantastic years, full of unexpected opportunities and disappointments. Never in my wildest dreams would I have anticipated the ups and downs, the joys and the frustrations – but overall the fun and friendship.

The demands of Silverfit and its sustainability were evermounting – with all the publicity and everyone wanting a Silverfit session near them, wherever they lived. Achieving that expansion is a serious challenge. The Silverfit formula is successful, and the opportunities to get funding for delivery of sessions to get local older communities more active and less isolated are there, but funding for core management remains significantly absent. In our most recent applications, some funders have agreed to support our instructors and venue hire, but rejected core costs, including all the valuable data analysis we do, proving the long-lasting health value of Silverfit sessions for older individuals and in saving money for the NHS and social care. But we remain optimistic that, with our weekly attendance averaging 455 Silverfitters, and counting our detailed statistical evidence on over 1260 older

people with an average age of sixty-eight, that we will be able
to prove the benefits of an organisation run by older people
for older people, with our sandwich formula of socialising,
activity and more socialising, and an emphasis on getting
the message out that it is never too late to start. Surely there
is a sponsor out there with a vested interest in fitter, happier oldies?

As the CEO, working sixty hours plus each week, I was
still a volunteer, and with a great but small paid team behind
me. I believe passionately in the cause, I have met some fantastic new friends and we all know that physical activity is
essential for healthier ageing. Whenever I go to one of the
venues, Silverfitters seek me out to tell me just how much
difference it has made to their lives. They feel more confident, have less pain and more friends, visit doctors less, and
the Silverfit sessions are key dates in their week. They are
of course becoming more active, and this active lifestyle is
extending way beyond one session as they join new friends
for a weekend walking, a silver cheerleading event or a walking football match. And they keep coming. Our increasing
evidence is showing that most participants remain active for
over a year in comparison to exercise on referral systems,
where people join a Lycra-clad gym for a limited time. In
these cases, research indicates that activity levels tail off very
quickly and many return to inactivity. Above all, I know and
can see Silverfitters are having fun. How do you measure the
number of smiles on people's faces as they warm up together
or practise a new silver-cheerleading routine to Billy Joel's
'Uptown Girl', waving their pompoms and strength training
at the same time? Our cheerleaders are being invited to an
increasing number of events, including a silver cheerleading
demonstration before the Duke of Kent, in front of the hal-
lowed altar of Southwark Cathedral, to the loud music of Phil

Collins and the lyrics of 'Can't Hurry Love'. We loved every minute of it, and the Duke clapped enthusiastically.

In terms of my own sports, my confidence level was higher after the Vichy Ironman in August 2015. Arguably it was too high. Yet again, along with Steve, I had signed up for another Ironman Lanzarote, determined to finish this time. So there I was, back on the island on 20 May 2016, registering again, surrounded by so many friends and Lanzarote residents wanting this old woman to have another go and not get stopped after 100k on the bike.

So yet again, at 7 a.m. on the Saturday morning I was down on the beach, right at the back of the huge gang of wetsuited bodies, for the final countdown. Then I was chased down into the water and off on the swim, out to the first buoy, and then turning left along the long row of buoys parallel to the beach. There weren't as many fish to marvel at this year and as I turned at the far point, back towards the start, I could see the final buoy, some eight hundred metres away, and that unmistakable, huge logo of the Hotel Fariones. It is so easy to sight on, that even I as one of the poorest of the swimmers wondered how anyone could not go in a straight line. But as I slowly approached it, I was tired, drained, and for the first time ever I began to doubt my ability to get out of the water, run the that familiar couple of metres up the sandy beach, around a bend and plunge back into the water for another 1900-metre swim.

My doubts increased over the last two hundred metres, and as I reached the sandy bank, I could see my fellow competitors ahead of me stepping slowly back into the water. Gone was the speed and excitement of their first entry. They looked as hesitant as I felt. Yet more demoralising was the endless stream of swimmers who had finished both laps and were running up the beach, unzipping wetsuits as they made their way to their bikes. The leaders had gone that way ages before, and as I mounted the beach, something deep inside asked 'Why? Can you really do it this year? After 100k of hard riding you failed to meet the cut-off on the bike last year. Can this year be any different? You are knackered, you aren't up to it.' To the consternation of all the marshals, cheering spectators and the Green Team from Club La Santa, so loyal in their support of me, I conceded I just couldn't do it. I was quitting.

Excuses, excuses – since then, I have reflected long on that second failure in Ironman. Was it a lack of confidence after the previous experience? Was it a lack of effective training? I had put in the hours and done the sessions that Annie had prescribed, but maybe not at the intensity required or in the right state of mind or body when I was working such long hours on Silverfit. Just recently I had cause to look back at some contentious, undoubtedly stress-inducing emails and spreadsheets I had written and I realised they were all sent the day before that Ironman race, from my hotel room in Lanzarote. Any other sane competitor would have been chilling on the beach, ensuring adequate nutrition and relaxing. Or maybe, the big one, this old woman's body really is getting old and it can't any more.

But that negativity and self-doubt has almost been drowned by the increasing media interest in Silverfit and my status as the founder. Fortunately the media focus was still based on my success in the Vichy Ironman, and me as the oldest British woman to do it. That is, of course, nowhere near the achievement of Sister Madonna Buder. She has completed forty-five Ironman triathlons and finished Ironman Canada at the age of eighty-two. Perhaps God was on her side. Or, as she put it when asked about her training: 'My coach is the Man upstairs; and, also, He gave me a body to listen to.' What an inspiration to us all.

More fun lay ahead, and in July 2016, still smarting from the Ironman debacle, I was off again to what has become an annual extended-family event: the New York City Triathlon. I had discovered that Billy Joel was doing a concert at Madison Square Garden three days before the tri, so I went over early. Gary and two of his colleagues from Navig8 reluctantly joined me, and we had a fantastic evening. Starting with a costly bottle of bubbly, we had a great supper. I was the only one of the group anxious to leave the restaurant, to get to Madison Square Garden and avoid missing a single moment. After all, Billy Joel had been my sole companion, cycling all my 880-mile share of Race across America. Then, suddenly I slipped or tripped up on the pavement. High heels flying, I went crashing to the ground on my right side. There was blood everywhere. The bad grazing was all up my right arm, the right of my forehead and my right calf. However, I was back on my feet instantly and heading for the concert. As we reached the queue wending its way up the stairs towards the ticket inspection, I was oblivious of the awful and bloody sight I presented. Fortunately, whilst I queued two of the guys, acutely embarrassed, disappeared to find a local pharmacy. They returned with a range of bandages and plasters to cover the mess and in we went.

It was a fantastic concert – the bandages, clearly evidencing my fragility, enabled me to push my way to the front of all the standing, cheering crowds in the circle. Billy Joel was absolute magic singing 'Keeping the Faith', 'Make You Feel My Love', 'Piano Man' and even 'Uptown Girl'. Tony Bennett joined in for his ninetieth-birthday celebration to sing 'New York, New York'. I felt no pain at all, just a slight muscle/tendon discomfort in my upper arm, but I put that down to my cheering and arm-waving exuberance with such magic, familiar songs. That night, I did a few stretching exercises for my sore arm and slept soundly.

Kate, who was by now at Heathrow and on her way to New York, had heard what had happened. On the phone she insisted, 'Mum, get it X-rayed.' 'No,' I assured her, 'its only muscle.' 'Mum, get it X-rayed,' she repeated. I said I would get it done when I got back to the UK four days later. 'Mum' – yet again – 'get it done today. It will show more now than if you leave it till you get home.' Finally, though confident it was all superficial grazing, with a slight muscle strain, I agreed and cheerfully found a local clinic.

After the X-ray the consultant came back into the room carrying a soft black sling. 'I am sorry to tell you that you have fractured your shoulder, and you need to keep your arm in this sling for several weeks, restricting the mobility as much as you possibly can.'

Later Kate told me that it was a very common but undiagnosed injury for mountain bikers. Like me, they assume it is just muscle or tendon injury in the upper arm, which leads to loads of normal mobility, rather than the essential immobilisation while the shoulder bone heals. A powerful message to all cyclists. Never throughout the next weeks did I feel any pain in my shoulder, despite the broken bone there.

I realised that I couldn't race, so I joined Kate and Jane on the sidelines as spectators. We were the New York City Triathlon support team. That was fun. As our team members jumped off the platform into the Hudson, I felt no envy at all. We sipped a glass of wine while they were out on the bike, all in their high-viz pink T-shirts we had brought from the UK. But there was a tinge of envy as we all sat together in a bar after the race, celebrating their successes and comparing their times.

Julian Robertson, one of our team, whom I had known since he was a ten-year-old badminton player in Northamptonshire, and who had subsequently played in three Olympics, was one of the GB Badminton coaches who was going off, two days later, to the Rio Olympics. What a wonderful experience and what a privilege. Could it really be as great as 2012 in London? I had watched so many events in London and I was really envious. 'Well, I think I can get you some badminton tickets,' Julian said. My son Gary followed up by offering some of his air miles, and suddenly it was a reality. I was off to Rio, on my own, my arm in the sling, a week or so later.

Again, another of those small, unplanned events shaped the whole experience. Walking down Camden High Street a few days later, I saw a smallish Union Jack. A eureka moment dawned – Kate sewed the GB flag onto my black sling and the real fun started.

Full of trepidation, I arrived in Rio on day six of the Olympics. I was very aware of the political issues of hosting the Olympics, the financial problems linked to the massive budget deficit, corruption allegations, people forced out of their homes to build venues, and the threat of the Zika virus. I was also aware of the huge police and military presence, clearly influenced by recent terrorist events worldwide. Like most visitors, I was confused at the beginning by planning journeys in the huge size of Rio and the Olympic area and the considerable distance between the main venues. Even the transfer from one Rio airport to another was followed by a very long cab ride to my first hotel, at Barra Beach.

The next morning I awoke to the most beautiful seaside view and I was off to watch Team GB at the badminton. What an adventure. I ordered a cab to the venue at Riocentro, which was close to but not part of the new Olympic Park. All too soon we began to experience the long traffic jams of the Rio transport system. For mile after mile the heavy traffic crawled along the modern three-lane dual carriageways. For long periods we were stationary. The inside lanes was sectioned off with a concrete kerbs for the fabulous bendy buses. With the lane to themselves, they pulled in every mile or so at newly designed stations for passengers to alight.

Worse was to come in my cab. We reached a police cordon as we approached the Olympic Park. Private vehicles were denied access. Assuring me it was at least a 5k walk, the driver reversed and went on around an effective ring road, to try to get into the next entrance into the Olympic Zone, again without success. It was third time lucky when finally, at my insistence, he dumped me at another 'forbidden entry', some 3k from Riocentro. It had proved to be a very expensive cab ride.

I set off walking towards the Rio 2016 Olympic Games. I was having fun, smiling at every passer-by as I walked, oh so safely, my GB sling to the fore. I went past the entrance to the athletes' village where a mass of GB bikes were being unloaded. Was that Cav? I wasn't sure, but I waved and wished them all the best. Finally, I was approaching the venue, with the badminton hall, boxing arena, table tennis and more. The queue to get in was long. As I approached, it was airport security at its tightest. I had been promised there would be a ticket from the GB team waiting for me inside, and with only my passport, proof of hotel accommodation, old age and GB sling I sailed through security without a ticket in my hand.

Then, after a quick text and a reflection on the miracles of modern technology, there was Julian to greet me, enjoy a cup of coffee between the team's games and give me some more badminton tickets. Over the next few days I saw loads of the badminton. I soon learnt that once inside most of the venues, you could sit where you wanted, regardless of seat numbering. But whoever was playing on those three courts, it was badminton at its very best – the rallies, the strategic positioning and above all the pace of the shuttlecock – often faster than 200mph – which was highlighted on screens for all to see.

I saw Gabby and Chris Adcock win their match, and marvelled at their complementary skills, their partnership, caring support and encouragement. Was their aim to be the first married couple to win gold since 1920? I also saw the match they finally lost, knocking them out of the competition, and I cried for them. How heartbreaking to train for so long, to come so far, to have such high national expectations on them and then to lose. How, I wondered, do they recover? I asked Julian how he and the other coaches help rebuild them. 'We reminded them how well they played and pick out all the positives from the match,' he said. 'We have kept motivational clips from that match and also others leading in to the games. Fun and banter come hand in hand and this breaks the ice of disappointment. Rest and recovery, then on to practice. Anything that can be taken out of the match they lost can be used to learn from.' Inspirational advice I need to take on board.

I watched Julian and another of the coaches sitting in the corner of the court for each match, impassive for the most part but advising their athletes at every break or change of ends. I felt so proud to know them and be part of such an intimate family feeling – waving my GB flag, wearing my necklace of GB flowers and with my GB sling in front. I loved it. I watched Marcus Ellis and Chris Langridge win their men's doubles matches, getting to the quarter finals and then, in a brilliant match, reaching the semi-finals. Again, it was the thrill of watching their interaction, their seamless play as a doubles pair – playing to individual strengths. The boys delivered a fantastic bronze medal, the first in men's doubles ever for Team GB.

Interestingly, two sides of the three-court stadium were absolutely packed, but on the other side were the empty areas for the media and the corporates. But it was great to see the other athletes watching and cheering their colleagues on. Andy and Jamie Murray came to watch, so did Sir Steve Redgrave and Denise Lewis, all cheering and waving GB flags. The athletes tended to know each other well and were sharing accommodation in the same quarters of the athletes' village.

But it was sad that the media and cameras in so many venues often seemed to focus on the empty seats of that corporate and media reserved area. It gave a slightly false picture of Rio 2016, although at the beginning, seats were too expensive for the local community.

After my first badminton session I went off to explore the big world of the Rio Olympics. Out past the flags of the approach to Riocentro, and less than a mile down the main road, was the huge Bus Rapid Transport (BRT) station – the main bendy bus station. There, for the first time, I experienced the fabulous welcome of the Olympic volunteers. They were so, so proud to be there. Apparently they had been selected from over a quarter of a million applicants. Many had a big badge with their name and 'I speak English' on it. They were all keen to ask what I thought of Brazil. Did I like their country, was it as good as the London Olympics and did I live in London?

It was one of the volunteers who confidently explained the brilliance of their new BRT network, which had just been completed. These fast buses were linked to the newly extended metro system and the railways. Their Rio transport strategy had recognised the massive cost to their society of all those wasted hours in endless traffic jams and the dangerously toxic fuel emissions. So, they told me, the Olympics and the World Cup had provided the incentive to transform their public transport system. Memorably, one of them so, so proudly told me it was free to me, as an 'older person', and that I should take advantage. 'You must,' he insisted, 'go on the BRT bus back to your hotel at Barra Beach. It is just one change of BRT bus. Just follow the crowds and it runs late into the night.' They warned me to take care at the railway stations, but assured me I was safe on the BRT system. They sounded more dubious about cab drivers.

Before trying the transport system out, I walked on down to the Olympic Park, with the velodrome, the tennis courts, the two aquatics centres with the diving and many other sporting venues, though not the athletics stadium, which was many miles away. I heard the roars of the crowd as I went past the tennis stadium, only realising later it was Andy Murray winning the final and his gold medal. And then, for the first time, I started to see all the box offices at each venue, temporary buildings often with four to six volunteers at individual windows. Some had an 'I speak English' card. They were selling tickets to all the venues, so again, with the production of my passport or my driving licence I was able to get more tickets. I will never know how or why I came to have my driving licence with me, but it proved absolutely invaluable. I would show it at every box-office window, and it was half price for a senior.

The computerised ticket system was very efficient. I found out, from the woman in front of her electronic ticketing screen in the box office, that I had purchased the last available public ticket to see Jason Kenny and Cav in the velodrome. Every single volunteer went out of their way when they saw my sling and GB flag, to get me a seat at the front. The fact, too, that I was an older woman on my own led to a gentle protectiveness. Their enthusiasm was infectious; I revelled in the fun and enjoyment, and their pride in Brazil.

For the first time, I entered one of the multi-event venues, and around several seating areas in the centre of the various venues I saw some of the numerous café and snack cabins. The queues were long and they only stocked a range of Coca-Cola products and Skol beer. Burgers were the staple food on offer, and apart from the occasional stall that did offer some Brazilian meatballs and the odd salad, there was no healthy food to purchase. The link between the pinnacle of sport, the Olympic Games, and the main sponsor, Coca-Cola, is ironic, particularly in the light of the current UK debate on the link between sugary drinks and obesity with all the subsequent chronic risks.

To my frustration, I only bothered to bring back three of the now sought after beer cups as souvenirs – a unique design for each sport. I was totally unaware they were to become collector's items and that many people were buying drinks, only to throw the beer away and keep the sport-specific plastic cups.

The velodrome, with huge screens at either end, appeared identical to London's. By getting to the front, I could literally feel the wind as Laura Trott raced by, less than a metre away from me. I watched her winning two gold medals and then after her race, Union Jack around her, she came over to talk to her family only a few metres away. I also saw her sitting in the middle, anxiously watching a screen in front of her, when Jason Kenny was racing in the Keirin, with that guy on the motorbike – the Derny – leading the riders out for the first seven laps. Faster and faster until they are at 50kph and the Derny leaves the track and they race their final two laps. But challenges followed. Had Kenny overtaken the Derny slightly too early? A long wait ensued, before he was exonerated and the race began again.

The rules of the omnium were bafflingly obscure. I saw at

close range that awful swerve of Cav down the track slope that led to the mega crash and the serious injury of his Korean rival. But what a privilege to see so many GB golds being won on my four separate visits to the velodrome and to hear the national anthem being played so often.

I missed seeing the diving pool turning green, but did see Jack Laugher diving for gold, and saying subsequently that he thought it could be ink from advertising hoardings leaking into the water. I had chosen to miss Tom Daley's qualifying dives one morning, as I went to another event in different venue. I was so confident that by booking a seat for the afternoon session I would see him diving for the medals. I was astounded that he didn't make the final and disappointed I had missed some of his brilliant high-scoring dives in the morning.

On another day, I was in the aquatics centre, watching the semi-finals of the water polo, wishing I fully appreciated the rules. I certainly admired the superb acceleration and swimming skills of those players.

Many of the athletics events were very late at night, leading to slightly less comfortable journeys and more complicated changes of transport. The athletics stadium was served by the main line railway and not the BRT so it necessitated a longish walk from the rail station to the BRT bus station. Mo Farah wouldn't be racing until gone midnight one night, so I gave that one a miss. However, I watched his 10k from high up in the stadium. He overtook the field, just below me, to race the last two hundred metres for gold. I am sure it coincided with Greg Rutherford doing the long jump below.

The hockey was another highlight. I wasn't sure that I wanted to travel all the way to yet another far-flung venue, but Team GB was in the final and as an old friend of mine once said, 'The best of anything is worth watching.' It was a thrilling experience. Maddie Hinch was the highlight. Without her brilliant goalkeeping throughout the match, GB would never have able to conclude with a draw and the memorable final penalty shootout against the Netherlands. I was so lucky to be at the front of the corner of the end they had the shootout and watched this talented twenty-seven-year-old goalkeeper managing to block every single goal attempt from the Dutch team, securing the gold medal for Great Britain. She looked so chunky in all of her padding and I was staggered when I saw her, months later, in a celebration in Trafalgar Square, a glamorous, slim athlete.

Best of all was one night in the athletics stadium. I was near the front, overlooking the tunnel that the athletes come through into the stadium. Not visible to cameras or the public, I could see Usain Bolt chatting in the tunnel, so clearly relaxed and sociable with the other athletes before the 4 × 100 relay. And then his final leg of the relay started just in front of me. He was the ultimate showman: whilst others were tensely crouching, Usain was still joking. Then finally as the race started, he was down – and wow – he won.

Despite my frequent attendance at various box offices, I had not managed to get a ticket for the triathlon. The tickets that enabled holders to go down onto the beach and along-side the cycle and run tracks remained 'sold out'. I tried at the box office the night before, to be told yet again that there were no tickets left. Early the next morning, happening to be wearing my bright pink New York City Triathlon T-shirt, I went for a slow jog along Copacabana Beach. The sling prevented any speedy running as I went along the beach to the box office that I knew opened at eight to join the queue at around 7.30 a.m.

At about ten to eight a man came up to our queue and asked me if I wanted a ticket. 'What for?' I asked. 'The

triathlon,' he replied. 'Oh, yes please, how much?' 'Nothing,'
he said, 'they are two family tickets.' He gave one to me and
the guy next to me in the queue the other. I naively and perhaps rudely asked 'Who?' and he replied that he would sooner
not say. It was only as he went away that others in the queue
said, 'I'm sure he is the Brownlees' dad.' I rushed after him to
say thank you again and what a fantastic job he and his wife
had done as parents – managing that level of competition and
also loyalty between brothers as they achieve such incredible
sporting heights, and have lifted the sport of triathlon to
another level. And how thoughtful to enable someone in the
queue to benefit from the tickets they had been allocated.

A couple of hours later, with only a few of the real VIPs
in front of me, the triathletes came right past as they went to
line up on the beach, to be introduced individually and then
for the magic of the swim start. It was only an unbelievable
seventeen minutes later – compared with my forty-five minutes – that the first competitor emerged from the water to
mount the sandy bank to transition. Watching the eight laps
of the bike, the Brownlee brothers were close together at the
transition, dropping their bikes and helmets and racing out on
the run. I was cheering madly as Alistair, closely shadowed
by Jonny, finally came down the finish straight for gold and
silver, both collapsing to the ground and hugging each other.
The tears really streamed as they mounted the podium for
their medals and our national anthem played. How proud
their parents must be, and what a fantastic job the Brownlees
have done for the sport.

The afternoon of the women's triathlon, I was opposite
the stand where both Non Stanford's and Vicky Holland's
families were anxiously watching. What an incredible finish
for two friends, teammates who had trained together and
lived in the same flat, with the bronze medal decided by such

a close margin. Opposite me, one mum put her head down, the other was cheering – what an ordeal for any family. I had been there, anxiously watching Gary in international tournaments, and could identify with their emotions.

As I left all the excitement and walked along Copacabana Beach with my suitcase to change hotels – they all had such limited space – approaching me was Annie Emmerson, who had been commentating on the triathlon. She was with Sarah Richardson, who had produced the BBC film of me in 2013. Sarah was now responsible for producing several of the Olympic events and she needed to go back to her room, so Annie and I went off for coffee. Five minutes later, Sarah came rushing back: 'Annie, Dan Walker wants to interview Eddie – take her down to the beach TV studio now!'

It was a good kilometre further down the beach, and what fun it proved to be, in such a small, intimate tent-like structure on the sand. The producer talked to me casually for a few minutes, then pointed for me to sit alongside Dan and we both watched the hockey on the small screen in front of us – there were complications as the match had switched channels, Dan explained. Then suddenly we were live and just chatting. The sling, the flag, my age, links to Ironman, Silverfit as a source of INSPIRE and, most embarrassing of all, 'So you binned that crucial badminton bronze medal-decider match for the triathlon?' The odd interruptions from the beach just below and behind us were fun and I learnt how Dan had been invited to the wedding of the bride who, with her hen-party friends, had featured live on the BBC coverage the previous day. I had no idea our interview was going out at a peak UK evening time until the texts started pouring in, including from Julian, who was watching from the athletes' hall at the badminton venue.

And then to my final event, after sharing a couple of those

great but intoxicating Brazilian cocktails, caipirinhas, with Annie. I had a ticket for the beach volleyball final in the magnificent stadium further along the beach. It was late at night, the seat high, high up, but what a spectacle. It was Brazil versus Italy, before a sell-out local crowd. It poured and poured with rain and the volunteers came round with effective waterproofs for us all. It was a thrilling and incredible event that Brazil finally won, to the raucous approval of the local community.

It had been a wonderful end to a fantastic experience and somehow it seemed appropriate that on my last day, in the cab back to the airport, we were passing the marathon runners on their final 10k. I was left hoping that the billions spent on the construction of the BRT and extension and modernising of the Rio metro rail system would be as effective for their struggling economy as the development of east London has been for London.

Back to reality in the UK, and I immediately sought out Elaine, my physio. At some point, I reflected, I was going to have to come out of the sling. I saw a consultant who, after surveying the original X-rays, seemed genuinely surprised by my speed of recovery and range of movement. Clearly those weeks of immobility had been the perfect advice back in New York. And maybe the fact that I was still physically active, with all the benefits for bone and muscles. I still had problems, though, reaching out and up. I wondered if I would be able to swim again. Elaine yet again came to my rescue and gave me advice on strength training to increase the range of movement of my healing shoulder. I was totally compliant and every day I lifted those 1kg weights in all prescribed directions and to my joy I was able three months later to get back in the pool and stretch out as I crawled, albeit as slowly as ever, through the water.

In 2016, thanks to Sigma Sports, Steve and I found Zwift – an incredible high-tech solution to serious bike training in my own home, on a turbo. On a screen in front of me, I can see a figure with my name and the GB flag above it on a bike travelling through imaginary American islands called Watopia – the fabulous scenery, plus the ups and downs on the hills, and in real time other named riders alongside or overtaking me. The flags of their country identify the riders – early morning in the UK often has riders from the Far East and after lunchtime there is a surge of American riders. For me, the real joy twice a week is the Ride London route where I am happily cycling along the banks of the Thames, then up and around Victoria Memorial, Trafalgar Square and a timed sprint up the Mall. After an imaginary tunnel comes the real fun, the ascent of Box Hill, with only the flapjack in the café at the top missing. I feel so proud to have been one of the earlier UK riders even though I am too scared to join some of the team races. It was exciting one day to be 263rd on a time trial with Mark Cavendish up there as number one. And even better, one Sunday I was doing the 100k KISS (Keep It Simple Stupid) race along the roads of London, whilst my son was soaring up and down serious climbs in the Surrey Hills from his home and my grandson, on a third turbo at his house, was on a magic ride with Mark Cavendish leading the group. That was intergenerational sport at its best, with all three of us benefiting hugely from the training. And another opportunity is coming: to run on a treadmill along the same bike routes, my phone with the software in front of me. Incredible technology, making the most of games software, but offering effective, structured and efficient training.

I returned to London from Rio to learn of three incredible and totally unexpected awards. As usual, I attended the AGM of the Serpentine Running Club and to my amazement I was awarded life membership of the club that has given me so much. What a privilege.

Equally unexpectedly, I received a call from the Cabinet Office to tell me that they were planning to award me their Points of Light for volunteering and Silverfit. The daily Points of Light award recognises 'outstanding individual volunteers – people who are making a change in their community'. I was to be the 599th winner, on 31 October 2016, as 'Britain's oldest Ironwoman and the founder of the Silverfit charity to support older people to get fit'. I got a certificate and a lovely letter, signed by Theresa May: 'You have inspired thousands to get fit and healthy. Demonstrating with your own remarkable achievements that exercise is something everyone can enjoy throughout their lives.' WOW!

And finally, and totally out of the blue, the University of Nottingham awarded me an Excellence Award for Alumni and invited me to a presentation ceremony in mid-December. Coinciding with the presentation of degrees to several faculties, this event was the most emotional and gratifying. On arrival I was dressed in gown and hat. I learned, for the first time, that my floppy hat denoted my PhD. It was on 22 December 2016, the twenty-second anniversary of Phil's death, and tearfully I felt as though I was receiving it on behalf of Phil and myself. He, as the County Surveyor and County Planner/Architect of Nottinghamshire, merited it so, so much more, but the university had never had the time to recognise the achievement of their 1965 civil engineering graduate before he died. There I was, proudly on the stage with the Vice-Chancellor and three other award winners, my kids in the front row before me, as my sporting history and charity work was read out before I collected the trophy. Such a humbling experience. And then, following the award, we remained on stage, and clapped, and clapped, and clapped for hours as hundreds of students were individually presented with their degree certificates. That day I also learned that clapping gains far more steps in our competitive family Fitbit group than any other exertion.

As I reached the end of 2016 I was hesitating, yet again, about another Ironman. Was I really too old? Had I got the mental and physical capacity? Was I just being driven by the experience of failure? I asked Josie Perry of Performance in Mind what I would need to finish an Ironman and Annie about how she would guide the training. Josie said:

> Eddie has the fitness and technical skills she needs to finish an Ironman. And she absolutely has the tenacity – but she needs to give herself the best possible chance to be beat the cut-off times. In the build-up she needs to focus on herself and her goals. Eddie's role at the centre of so many projects means she risks getting distracted along the way. Specifically, she needs to focus in the pool so she completes the swim course comfortably and is able to get on the bike with time to spare. Overall, she is currently lacking the magic ingredient that makes everything in life feel easier: confidence. Following the training she has been set, taking advice from her army of expert friends, focusing on her swimming and reflecting upon the fact she has already completed two of the hardest Ironman courses in the world (Lanzarote and Kona) will give her that magic ingredient and yet another Ironman finish.

Annie also emphasised the mental issues of tackling another Ironman, this time at seventy-four years of age; her words were to prove remarkably accurate for 2017 too:

I've known you for eleven years now and you don't look any different from when I met you. It's all about confidence. Because you are older, you sometimes think you can't do as much. You've had ups and downs and a meltdown in Lanzarote, but that was all about your headspace. You have got to have the right headspace to do an Ironman. There was a lot going on for you outside of sport that affected you. It's keeping you positive and as the years creep by, you don't think that. At the moment there's no reason you can't do it. I don't see anything about you physically that has changed. The only thing is your commitment to Silverfit and just, generally, in life. It does make getting the miles in training difficult. But then sometimes you can say to yourself that if you overtrain, would that be any good for you? Is it the fact that you do have other things in your life that prevent you from overtraining? So I guess it is all about balance and you have just about got that balance now. I think you could probably go faster but then there are higher risks of injury. The fact that your life is balanced by having your family and Silverfit play big parts works in your favour more than you think it does. The challenges for me as your coach are more about giving you the confidence to know that you can still do it. I really believe you can do it and I am not just saying that because if as a coach you have doubts, you should say it. So yes, we just have to look after the knees a bit more. You had a shoulder injury but that was because you got pissed and fell over. That was absolutely nothing to do with ageing or wear and tear. The rest of your body is the same. So other than you worrying about your knees and having to protect them, the rest of the body and the engine is still the same and present no challenges for a coach.

Finally, I signed up for Ironman Frankfurt. Then on the penultimate day of 2016, I got an email from Dorothy, responding to my note in my Christmas card. An old Nottingham University friend, she told me she had been in her kitchen in Maastricht when she had got our note in a Christmas card to say that Phil was terminally ill. Fate or not, I went googling and realised that Ironman Maastricht had a slightly longer time limit, of 16 hours, 15 minutes. Yes! In went my transfer application, successfully. I just hoped that on 6 August 2017 I would hear the words 'You are an Ironman' as I came across the finish line. But despite Phil's encouragement somewhere up there, as we had both spent a lovely weekend with those friends when they lived in Maastricht, it was not to be!

In the interests of safety, they say, Ironman had created a new rolling start system. Instead of the mass starts and the dangers inherent in 1300 bodies rushing into the water together, everyone lines up to jump in one or two at a time, with chip timing measuring the entry point. Slower swimmers are asked to go at the back, and I was worried that the first cut-off on the bike, after 90k, was in real time: 2 p.m. Even if I could get out of the water within two hours I was going to have to push it really hard on the bike, half an hour faster than those who had lined up at the font of the line. It may be a safer system, but is surely discriminatory against us slower swimmers. The final cut-off, after 180k on the bike, was however based on my own chip time, and would come ten hours after I started.

Ever the conformist, I jumped in safely, having lined up with my cautiously anticipated two-hour swim time and started swimming. I was totally unprepared for the next ten minutes, as the relay-team swimmers came in behind me – over, under and around, aggressive arms wildly thrashing.

They knew they didn't have to do the bike or the run, and were there just for the swim, so could really go for it. It was scary until they had all gone past me and suddenly I was on my own, swimming happily under three historic bridges in the Maas River. A quick look at my Garmin indicated I had swum twelve hundred metres in a really fast time.

Unusually, I was really enjoying this swim, aware that a friendly canoeist was keeping a watchful eye on me. I knew that the route went down the river and around an island, and at the halfway point, we clambered out of the water, jogged a few metres across land and a timing mat, then back into the water. Only then did I realise just how slow I had been, my slowest swim time ever. So clearly my Garmin was not accurately recording open-water distances, and I had been relaxing and enjoying the swim far too much. There was only one competitor after me. I really, really swam as fast as I could for the second half.

The final hundred metres were tough. There was an oddly churning current and I was surrounded by countless boats and canoeists – the entire support crew nearing the end of their shift and waiting to get out of the water too. As I mounted the ramp, I gratefully turned to wave and thank them. I made the cut-off time – just – to rapturous applause as the commentator enthused about their very last swimmer and the oldest woman too.

Onto a fabulous bike ride – two 90k laps. As the last competitor on to the bike, I was led out by a personal motorbike escort. I knew I had to push it as hard as I could, up hills and racing downhill. By now, many of the faster riders were overtaking me on their second lap. The support outside all the houses, shops and bars was fantastic. This was followed by a peaceful, fabulous flat 15k along the Maas path. Despite the enthusiastic, inebriated support, I was keeping a close eye on my watch and speedo on my average time, aiming successfully to stay above 24kph as son Steve had advised and fearing that 2 p.m. cut-off, which made no allowances for the thirty-minute delay before I started the swim. I made it with ten minutes to spare and jubilantly set out on the second lap. But this time I was alone – the crowds had gone, though the drink stations were still open and welcoming to the end. I must have let my average pace slip just that little bit to 23.8 as I made eye contact with all those volunteers marshalling and thanked them. Or maybe I was just a bit tired. As I reached the end I knew a vehicle was just behind me, and that I was close to the ten-hour personal cut-off from the chip timing system that had started as I jumped into the water at the swim start. If I am a couple of minutes over, I reassured myself, I am sure they will let me through. I was totally unprepared for that formidable official at the gate to transition. 'No,' he said, 'you are finished. It is 5.49 and transition closed at 5.45 p.m. You are four minutes outside your ten-hour cut-off time.'

There was another girl just behind me and then two more athletes who had been picked up by the sweep vehicle joined us. Just four minutes late after ten hours? I could not believe it. Despite our requests, he refused to let us discuss his decision with a race manager. Had he let us through, I had six hours and eleven minutes to do the marathon before midnight – I could walk it in that time. OK, rules are rules, but late by just 0.0066 per cent of the total time? I appreciate that road closures are very costly, and there was the need to open the roads at 5.45 p.m., but we had been off the main road for several minutes too.

Did I need a final blow? After a couple of congratulatory drinks with my son Steve, I loaded my bike onto the white van, SHIP MY TRI BIKE, NIRVANA emblazoned on the side, to be transported back to the UK. That night, the van was broken into and all ten of the Ironman racing bikes were stolen – 'TAKE MY TRI BIKE, NIRVANA?' Many weeks later I was still awaiting an insurance offer on my prized, comfortable and rare DeVinci bike.

So again I had mega unfinished business, albeit a good story. And yet again, the dilemmas resurfaced. Is this old body up to it? Maastricht had been going to be my last Ironman, my knees had their limitations and RAAM, and the eleven-year anniversary for the Serpentine Golden Girls, looms.

Again I was reminded of Julian's badminton advice and consolation to Chris and Gabby Adcock, as well as Josie Perry's thoughts:

> When you have set your sights on a race, put everything into it and it doesn't go to plan it can be really demoralising. In the few weeks after a disappointing event, athletes first need to grieve the race they wanted, then to analyse why their race didn't go the way they hoped and finally to make an action plan to put right their disappointment. For some, that will be quitting, but this risks having a nagging feeling forever of 'what if'. Eddie's approach of finding another Ironman is a great move. To do well at this race Eddie needs to make sure she really boosts her confidence. We get our most robust confidence from knowing we have the skills to do well and knowing we have been successful in the past. This means Eddie needs to remind herself about the skills and strengths she has and how they will help her in this race. She also needs to look back over her previous races and pull out elements of each (such as a fast bike ride on a course similar to this one) which highlight why she will be able to succeed in this Ironman.

The next week, in August 2107, I started to think about finding another Ironman with a slightly longer cut-off. Steve Trew had already laid the seeds. He was going to be the commentator of Ironman Cozumel in Mexico, and he had enthused about the venue, the Mexican culture and the race. I started to do my homework. After the bike theft, I would have to purchase a new bike and get used to it. The bike route was a flat but windy three-lap course but it was the swim that was unique, a point-to-point 3.8k ocean swim with a current behind, over coral reefs and aquatic life, but with unpredictably choppiness. Could I try once more? It took me just a few days to decide – Cozumel here I come!

And this time, despite competing demands, I did prioritise my training. For three months I conformed, indeed arguably over-conformed, to Annie's' programme. I swam more than eight or nine kilometres a week and really listened to Dan's advice: 'Chin down, elbows up for the catch, push back and rotate.' Thanks again to the GLL Sports Foundation award, I combined Silverfit sessions with swimming in the fantastic 50-metre pool at Crystal Palace. Twice I did an unbelievable 152 lengths of the 25-metre Brixton Rec pool on a Friday night, thinking of all those happy people outside enjoying the real nightlife of Brixton. I attended most of the Swim for Tri sessions with that horrendously early start at Mile End. Swim coaches at Serpentine Running Club did their best in Monday-night sessions. I continued some spin classes and did Zwift sessions almost every day, focused on building my strength. As Elaine had advised, I kept my running to a minimum, but with thanks again to the life membership that the Gym Group had given me, I regularly undertook her recommended strength training routines for my legs and loved the occasionally run along the Thames, the Serpentine handicap race or Burgess Park Parkrun.

I arrived in Cozumel confident I had done as much as possible. The hotel was fantastic, with great food and many other competitors staying there, as well as Steve Trew, his wife Von and his fellow commentators. Some factors would be beyond my control – high winds or, worst of all, a very choppy sea – but I was unusually calm. I was reading two books that helped the mental equilibrium: Chrissie Wellington's *To the Finish Line*, which had some great advice from such an authoritative professional triathlete's viewpoint; and *Redemption: From Iron Bars to Ironman*. I had heard John McAvoy speak a few weeks earlier at a conference, and had bought his book, partly to check out whether I had failed him as a social worker when he said he grew up in Lambeth, and spoke of the Walworth Road and armed robbery culture. In fact I had been working there long before he was born! But his history demonstrated so vividly the power of sport and physical activity to change lives, albeit that his incredible indoor rowing, biking and tread-milling achievements were all within Her Majesty's hospitality, then in 2013 he too became an Ironman.

And so, on race day, I was healthily apprehensive but positive. Zone3 had sponsored me with a tri-suit, and also a skinsuit for the swim – every second counts in resistance to the water – and the spirit amongst competitors was inspiriting: we were all in it together. So, having positioned myself towards the back of the rolling swim start, I finally went over the timing mat and plopped into the water. One day I must learn to dive! After the initial two hundred metres of turbulent cross-currents the swim was brilliant, with relatively little churn. The fish were fantastic, the countless volunteers on paddleboards and canoes so encouraging, and within an amazingly short time the two wooden structures came into view, behind which I had learned from the previous day's practice swim lay the enclosed area in which one could swim

with the dolphins. Finally I clambered out to see Steve and
Xavier on their mikes, shouting encouragement and com-
menting on my faster than anticipated time. Had I really
completed an Ironman swim in 1 hour, 32 minutes?

As I stripped off my new skinsuit and grabbed my bike I
was on cloud nine. And then, I heard the voice of my son
Steve, and Zwift expert, behind me: 'You need to average
25k an hour, Mum. Leave as much time as you can to walk
the run and minimise the damage to your knees.' I loved it:
I gave it my best, I rejoiced in the difference Zwift had made
to my biking strength and kept a constant eye on my pace.
I overtook many, but one rider in particular would pass me
back. And we yo-yo'd several times. The 10k towards the
south of the island was more isolated and windy, but I was
sustained by the incredible ocean views and many of the faster
guys overtaking me and shouting encouragement. It is tough
in a three-lap race as you reach the end of a 60k lap and those
strong athletes are going down the finisher straight, but for
me it was a left turn and back out on another lap. What fun,
though, with the exuberant local community out to support
in huge numbers, and great Mexican music pounding out,
or drummers performing from countless sources around the
route, the clappers, the bilingual encouragement in Spanish
and English: 'You've got it!' Had I really?

And finally, after 180k, I too turned into cheering crowds
along the finish straight. I dismounted, my bike taken by a
welcoming volunteer, then shoes changed and off on the run,
initially through lively urban Mexican life. I knew my time
was better than previously, and for the first time I began to
feel I could do it! Hundreds of times I returned high-fives
to youngsters proffering their hands, and it was going well.
But alert as ever to the frailty of my knees, I started to walk
the third lap. Then, with 7k to go, someone came alongside.

I recognised her as the cyclist who had shared much of the bike ride with me. We started to chat: Lynne came from the USA, and we talked about our families and our racing experiences, then realised we were both long-standing social workers. The last 5k slipped by as we compared remarkably similar experiences and client groups. With the miles marked along the route, and her Garmin measuring our pace, we were increasingly confident we would make the midnight cut-off. And as we neared the end, people in crowds again shouted 'You've got it!' Fantastic.

And then finally into the light of the finish gantry, to hear my good friend Steve Trew: 'Eddie Brocklesby, at seventy-four years the oldest woman, all the way from London, you are an Ironman. YOU ARE AN IRONGRAN!'

AFTERWORD

So I am still the lucky one; physically and mentally strong enough to make the most of my life, and being in a position to take on crazy challenges well into retirement has, I hope, played a small part in raising the profile of healthier, happier ageing, encouraging older people to be Silverfit.

Recalling the words of my granddaughter, 'The book should be called Madgran.'

I leave you with the fourteen lessons that my seventy-four years of life have taught me:

1. Staying healthy isn't rocket science: eat well and move more
2. It is never too late to find out what is important to you
3. If you want to stay mentally healthy then exercise – running was my survival
4. Exercising with others makes it easier and more enjoyable
5. Find your niche and the world is your oyster
6. Things rarely go the way you think they will: expect the unexpected

7. Dreams don't always live up to your expectations
8. Perception is everything: if you don't like something change it, if you can't change it then change your perception
9. Age is just a number
10. Take every opportunity to inspire and encourage others
11. Blood is thicker than water
12. Your health is your most valuable asset
13. Cope with failure and adversity and set a new goal
14. Keep moving onwards and upwards

ACKNOWLEDGEMENTS

My son Steve suggested *Irongran* – claiming limited memory of his childhood, so needing a written reminder! But he has been my Iron inspiration and mentor.

I have received massive help from so many others:

- Josie Perry, who guided and supported *Irongran* from the beginning.
- Members of all my sports clubs, originally South Notts Athletic Pacers, then Serpentine Running Club. They have provided the invaluable support and friendships that have sustained me, including our RAAM team of Serpentine Golden Girls and our priceless crew. Specific thanks to Manuel and Jan, who have permitted me to record their inspirational stories of overcoming adversity.
- My physio Elaine who, after the advice of Professor Haddad, inspired me, insisting that despite my injuries and chronic knee problems I could still compete, as long as I followed her instructions.
- Coaches Frank Horwill, Brian Welsh, Annie Emmerson, Dan Bullock and Steve Trew, and members of the Green Team at Club La Santa, all

of whom have tried, against the odds, to improve
the swimming, running and cycling technique of
this old woman.

- The Gym Group have given me life membership,
and GLL/Better have granted me their Sports
Foundation awards, enabling all those spin classes
and strength-training sessions.

- My co-founders, co-directors and funders of
Silverfit have supported me throughout and
facilitated the fun and friendship of all our
Silverfitters, who have proved it is never too late to
change inactive or isolated lifestyles.

- Paul Sinton-Hewitt and all at Parkrun,
that brilliant concept which influenced the
development of Silverfit.

- All those race organisers and volunteers, and
Zwift, who have made the journey possible, and
British Triathlon, who featured this old woman as
'This Girl Can'.

- Victoria Marshallsay, my literary agent, introduced
me to the brilliant *Irongran* team within Little,
Brown, where I have had such fun working with
Zoe Gullen, Adam Strange, Ella Bowman and
Aimee Kitson.

- And finally to my late husband, Phil, who issued
that challenge: 'You could never run all the way
to Northampton, let alone a half marathon.' Since
his death, my kids, Steve, Gary and Kate, with
their partners Jane, Angela and John and their
kids Jake, Jodie, Ben and Tilly, have kept me on
the relatively straight and narrow – pink bubbly
notwithstanding. Without my family the fun of
being Irongran, or Madgran, would not exist.

PICTURE CREDITS